HISNF
25.00

D0909997

DISCARD

"When it comes to Hell, Dante Alighieri is the definitive tour guide. But for today's (and quite possibly tomorrow's) living hell, you'll want to take Ira Rosofsky's delightfully wry narrative along for the ride. He accomplishes what few authors are capable of—taking an unnerving topic and turning it into a book so enthralling you won't want to put it down. Indeed, it's a meditation worthy of Marcus Aurelius and Jerry Seinfeld."

—ANDREW D. BLECHMAN, author of *Leisureville: Adventures in America's Retirement Utopias*

"In *Nasty, Brutish, and Long*, Ira Rosofsky provides a rare glimpse into the hearts and minds of the aging. As a psychologist who has worked in nursing homes and an immensely talented and sensitive writer, he manages to find the perfect telling details to bring this often neglected world alive for the reader."

—GAIL KONOP BAKER, author of *Cancer Is a Bitch (Or, I'd Rather Be Having a Midlife Crisis)*

"In an intriguing combination of personal story, social commentary, and scientific observation, a psychologist lifts the veil on nursing homes. Ira Rosofsky's presentation—laced with sharp humor—treats us to the nursing home experience from the variety of these viewpoints. All who have had experiences with nursing homes—whether as residents, relatives of residents, or professionals—should read *Nasty, Brutish, and Long,* as should anyone interested in a penetrating view of how we as a society care for and care about those too frail or elderly to care for themselves."

—LAURIE STILLMAN, Director, Public Health Policy and Advocacy Center, The Medical Foundation

"*Nasty, Brutish, and Long* is as much about the last years of life and the meaning of existence during old age as it is about nursing homes. Ira Rosofsky's personal narrative—along with the tales of the elderly he treats—contributes to a picture of the author as a fully engaged human being who tells his story with style and humor. And the story has an insightful and sensitive perspective on issues as varied as psychotherapy, psychopharmacology, the institutionalization of the aged, and our inevitable mortality."

—DAVID HALL, former principal, Sonia Shankman Orthogenic School, University of Chicago

NASTY,

BRUTISH,

and LONG

ADVENTURES IN OLD AGE AND

THE WORLD OF ELDERCARE

IRA ROSOFSKY

AVERY

a member of Penguin Group (USA) Inc.

New York

Published by the Penguin Group

Penguin Group (USA) Inc., 375 Hudson Street, New York, New York 10014, USA • Penguin Group (Canada), 90 Eglinton Avenue East, Suite 700, Toronto, Ontario M4P 2Y3, Canada (a division of Pearson Canada Inc.) • Penguin Books Ltd, 80 Strand, London WC2R 0RL, England • Penguin Ireland, 25 St Stephen's Green, Dublin 2, Ireland (a division of Penguin Books Ltd) • Penguin Group (Australia), 250 Camberwell Road, Camberwell, Victoria 3124, Australia • (a division of Pearson Australia Group Pty Ltd) • Penguin Books India Pvt Ltd, 11 Community Centre, Panchsheel Park, New Delhi–110 017, India • Penguin Group (NZ), 67 Apollo Drive, Rosedale, North Shore 0632, New Zealand (a division of Pearson New Zealand Ltd) • Penguin Books (South Africa) (Pty) Ltd, 24 Sturdee Avenue, Rosebank, Johannesburg 2196, South Africa

Penguin Books Ltd, Registered Offices: 80 Strand, London WC2R 0RL, England

Copyright © 2009 by Ira Rosofsky
All rights reserved. No part of this book may be reproduced, scanned, or distributed in any printed or electronic form without permission. Please do not participate in or encourage piracy of copyrighted materials in violation of the author's rights. Purchase only authorized editions. Published simultaneously in Canada

Most Avery books are available at special quantity discounts for bulk purchase for sales promotions, premiums, fund-raising, and educational needs. Special books or book excerpts also can be created to fit specific needs. For details, write Penguin Group (USA) Inc. Special Markets, 375 Hudson Street, New York, NY 10014.

ISBN 978-1-58333-336-5

Printed in the United States of America
10 9 8 7 6 5 4 3 2 1

BOOK DESIGN BY MEIGHAN CAVANAUGH

Neither the publisher nor the author is engaged in rendering professional advice or services to the individual reader. The ideas, procedures, and suggestions contained in this book are not intended as a substitute for consulting with a physician. All matters regarding health require medical supervision. Neither the author nor the publisher shall be liable or responsible for any loss or damage allegedly arising from any information or suggestion in this book.

While the author has made every effort to provide accurate telephone numbers and Internet addresses at the time of publication, neither the publisher nor the author assumes any responsibility for errors, or for changes that occur after publication. Further, the publisher does not have any control over and does not assume any responsibility for author or third-party websites or their content.

For Linda, Jonathan, Leah, Sammy,
and all our elders

CONTENTS

"My brother owns a nursing home in Lakewood, New Jersey, and the things he sees you could make a book out of. If somebody wrote it, it might do the world some good."

—PHILIP ROTH, *The Anatomy Lesson* (1983)

1 DO YOU PLAY CHESS?

Overture

Sam Rosen is telling me once again that he was married for seventy-seven years and suddenly he's all alone.

He is one hundred and two. A year ago, he was still living at home with his one-hundred-and-one-year-old wife. But at ancient ages your life expectancy is limited. She's buried in the cemetery. He's buried in the nursing home.

"Fit as a fiddle, and then she catches pneumonia! Then my kids sell the house and put me here. They don't even visit," Sam says.

"Seventy-seven years!" he reminds me.

He's sitting on his bed in the corner of a room considerably smaller than the average middle-class living room. I'm in a chair squeezed beside his bed. Books and magazines—most of them of a left-wing variety—are piled high on the nightstand. This small corner of the universe is all that is left to him after more than a century of living. It is no different from the small corners allotted to the hundred other residents of his nursing home or from the two million corners of similar rooms in the eighteen thousand nursing homes across our nation.

Two million out of a population of three hundred million may seem like a small number, but the nursing home experience will touch almost all. If you are sixty-five, your lifetime chances of spending time in a nursing home are 43 percent. If not you, it could be your parents.

As you age, your chances increase. Only 12 percent of people between sixty-five and seventy-four are in nursing homes, compared to one-third of those between seventy-five and eighty-four. If you live to eighty-five, your chances are better than one in two.

Sam defied the odds. For most of those seventy-seven married years, he lived in a big old Victorian house. It had only a few years on him. Queen Victoria died just a few years before Sam was born.

On the wall is a sepia photo of a cute couple.

"That's me and my wife," Sam tells me—the wife with a vintage bob; Sam with wavy hair, looking early Cagney.

Next to that photo is one of Sam, a lifetime later. He and the family are blowing out a one-hundred-candle cake. I idly wonder how they lighted the last candles before the first ones went out.

If you looked up *wizened* in the dictionary, there might be a picture of Sam. But he's ambulatory, can still read, and knows he's unhappy.

"Do you play chess?" Sam asks. "Or Scrabble?"

Every week I see him, I get this invitation along with a reminder that he was married for seventy-seven years.

The other day my daughter was flipping through the *Guinness Book of World Records*.

"What are you looking at?"

"I'm looking at the Longest, Daddy."

"Like what?"

"Well, the longest marriage was eighty-two years."

So Sam doesn't hold the record but still gets elected to the Marriage Hall of Fame.

I tell Sam I probably don't have time to play chess. I make a note to ask someone on the staff if they could play.

On the other bed, Ralphie, a mere child of eighty-four, is sitting on his bed flipping through sports magazines. I'm not sure Ralphie knows how to read as he looks mainly at the pictures of Alex Rodriguez, Michael Strahan, and Shaquille O'Neal, his radio tuned to the soul music station.

Ralphie, an African-American, and Sam, a Jew, are demographic anomalies in this largely Polish facility. Not that it doesn't happen, but I've never seen Ralphie or Sam with a visitor. For many of the Poles, if Mom can't be at home, the family will bring home to the nursing home—all the kids still arrayed around Mom, just like Sunday dinner. One younger woman, I thought she was on the staff, except she was a daughter sitting by her mom all day. The mother in her wheelchair holding a doll, the daughter wiping the drool off of Mom's perpetually smiling face.

Ralphie spent most of his life working construction, interrupted by a few years playing baseball in the Negro Leagues. "I took away a home run from Josh Gibson. Reached right over the fence. It was already gone." This might be the crowning point of his life. Occasionally, the staff tells me, one of his buddies comes by and they drive over to another nursing home to visit yet another buddy who has Alzheimer's. Then, in an act of defiance, he goes out for ice cream, fresh-made ice cream at the University dairy. It's poison to his diabetic body, already missing some amputated toes. For days, his blood sugar goes out of whack, but he bitterly complains about the lack of sweetness in his diet—and his life. He curses at the cook.

The cook won't speak to him. Why control your impulses when you're a dead man walking?

Ralphie is one of the never-married. He was living in subsidized senior housing, more or less not taking care of himself. They found him passed out with hyperglycemia following an ice cream binge. Someone wondered whether the flavor was Forbidden Chocolate. For Ralphie, landing in a nursing home is arguably landing on his toeless feet.

"I'd just as soon die if I can't have ice cream," he once told me.

Ralphie is in love with Gladys, another African-American.

Gladys sits most of the day in her wheelchair. A couple of strokes and she's mostly mute as tremors roll like waves through her body. She can hear us, and she struggles to respond in words that contort her lips into indescribable shapes before she collapses in frustration.

They say she's depressed.

Who can tell for sure?

Along with contraband ice cream, Ralphie lives for Gladys.

He's often wheeling her around. I wonder if she does more than tolerate him.

"When she dies, I'm out of here."

How far can he get? He walks with the stiff-legged Frankensteinian gait characteristic of those who can't bend their arthritic knees. He lurches from left to right as he totters forward.

Occasionally, a frustrated denizen of a nursing home will fly the coop, rolling off in a wheelchair or shuffling down the street pushing his walker before him. You could measure staff negligence by how far he gets. Typically, when caught, they'll say something like, "I really missed just having a beer." Or, "I was tired of being told when I could smoke." Or, "I was going to see my mother." The escapee might be eighty. Mom might be dead for thirty years.

The staff hates this stuff. Hours of paperwork and inquiries from the State.

Sam asks me again.

"Do you play chess?"

"Not very well," I answer this time.

Sam has told me his story many times. Aside from being married for seventy-seven years, as a very young man he led what appears to me as a romantic life in the nascent aviation industry. Flying his plane into a town, lifting the locals in the wild blue yonder for a dollar a ride. Things went bust in 1929.

Back in Connecticut, he married, scraped by, and started a small machine shop, something he learned from fashioning his own airplane parts. It was one of the thousands of shops that served Connecticut in its glory hard-core manufacturing days. He sidelined in radical politics.

"Did you ever hear of Paul Robeson? The singer? He was a friend of mine. Stayed at my house whenever he was in Connecticut."

Another story I've heard more than once sitting next to the latest copy of *The Nation* or *The Progressive*.

This time I get a variation on the theme.

"You know, I like to play chess. I like to play Scrabble, bridge, all the games. I taught my daughter cribbage. She was terrific. Hustled her way through college beating all the boys. I taught this one fellow to play chess and then I was going to be drafted for the war, but he was on the draft board. As a favor to me, I wasn't drafted."

I find it hard to reconcile his radical politics with draft avoidance during World War II. Maybe he's confused. After all, he was almost forty years old when we entered the war. Maybe he got a pass on the basis of his already advanced age nearly sixty-five years ago. Maybe they needed him at his machine shop building military

5

parts. Sam couldn't have been thinking about World War I. He was only twelve at the time.

"Seventy-seven years. I was married for seventy-seven years and now I'm here by myself," I hear again. "Can you imagine? Seventy-seven years! And here I am all alone. Do you play chess?"

We're interrupted. A nurse at the door. "I have something for you, Sam," she chirps.

Living in a nursing home is life interrupted. Your door is always open. The staff views closed doors with the suspicious eyes of a teenager's mother. But these people aren't sneaking joints or downloading porn. Walking down the hall on a typical morning, peering through the open doors, you see that they're mostly lying in bed—some eager for the staff to come, others hoping they won't bother.

Oblomov comes to mind, the hero of an 1858 Russian novel by Ivan Goncharov. On page one, Ilya Ilyich Oblomov is lying in bed—"in his dark-grey eyes there was an absence of any definite idea, and in his other features a total lack of concentration." Sounds like some of my case notes. On page 150, Oblomov gets out of bed. Idle and rich, Oblomov—living in the last decades of the czars—is superfluous, unproductive, and parasitical. There's little reason for him to get up. Nursing home residents—despite outward appearances—are hardly superfluous, unproductive, or parasitical. Their care and feeding is a $115 billion industry. We're not quite the Alaskan nomads who leave behind Old Koskoosh in Jack London's "The Law of Life." Old Koskoosh waits helplessly by his fire, dreaming of youthful hunts while the wolves circle in. Resigned and uncomplaining, he reflects, "Nature was not kindly to the flesh. She had no concern for that concrete thing called the individual. Her interest lay in the species, the race." In our supposedly humane culture, we keep our elderly alive as long as scientifically possible, and the eldercare industry profits from our humanity. Bottom line for me: if life expectancy were lower, or if it didn't so often end in a frail passage through the nursing home, I'd be in another line of work.

Looked at yet another way, the morning nursing home ritual is a parody of the levee of King Louis XIV. When the Sun King rose at eight-thirty each day, the first *valet de chambre* would pull the curtain surrounding the bed and announce, "It is time, Sire." Louis would open his eyes to a group of courtiers—each ready to play a precise role in his theatrical routine. In the nursing home, two or three aides enter the room and announce, "Time to get up, Joe." The aides draw the curtain around Joe and begin their morning routine. Attending the king, the first servant took hold of one of Louis's sleeves, the master of the bedchamber took the other, and they pulled off his nightshirt. These royal tasks imparted great prestige, fulfilled not by peasants but by high-ranking nobility. Louis liked to keep an eye on the opposition. He was an early adapter of Vito Corleone's leadership creed: "Keep your friends close, but your enemies closer." Joe's nursing home aides aren't thinking in terms of prestige or affairs of state. The aides' white outfits are an upwardly mobile improvement from the blue jackets of Wal-Mart. They'll get Joe dressed and deposit him in his wheelchair. Maybe they'll turn on his TV and pause for Jerry Springer before moving on to the next room. Louis would move on to be the King of France.

There is another parallel. Most of us flow between a public and private zone. We have at least one door we can close to the world. People in nursing homes have lost that door as, like Louis, they live their life in public.

———

The nurse at Sam's door is mixing up some crushed medicine in a little cup—the kind in which you get a side of cole slaw at the diner. She's on her med pass, another of the many daily routines. This is a landscape where the only spontaneity might be the screams of a person with not enough medication. All the routines are scrupulously documented. There is one set of books—procedure books—telling you what to do. There's another set of books—record books—in which you write down what you have done.

The nurse pushes a cart quite similar to the cart a flight attendant pushes down the aisle of an airplane. Many of the folks complain about the "service" as if they were in a bad hotel: "I ring this bell, but they never come." The top of the med cart is loaded with carefully counted medications. There are cups of water and tools to crush meds for the toothless or for those with swallowing problems. Orange juice or ginger ale is there for a chaser. Crushed meds are blended into applesauce. There are vile-tasting high-calorie health shakes to fatten up those with a "failure to thrive." This happens three shifts a day, one med pass per shift. Sometimes I'll ask a nurse for a favor and I'll get the response, "I'm in the middle of my med pass. Can you wait until I finish?" Residents—we try not to call them patients—ask a question or a favor and get the same answer: "Wait until I'm finished." The routines get the staff through the day. A med pass will get a nurse through at least an hour or two of her shift. And when she's doing her pass, she can't be interrupted.

For the staff, a day in the nursing home is like an industrial process. This is not a creative workshop but a place where every procedure is by the book—or, more accurately, every procedure is by one of the many books. These recipes bake no bread. The idea is not to come up with a product at the end of the shift, but to keep a body alive to pass on to the next shift that operates out of the same set of books.

One of the main processes is the process of medicating the residents. There's a long list of drugs: Zyprexa, Prozac, Lipitor, Remeron, Xanax, Coumadin, Ativan, Ambien, albuterol, Lexapro, Percocet, insulin, Celebrex, Celexa, Vioxx, Neurontin, Plavix, Risperdal—the pharmacopoeia of American medicine today—but no Viagra or Ortho Tri-Cyclen.

The elderly—whether in nursing homes or not—represent a license to print money for the pharmaceutical industry. The average nursing home resident ingests about ten drugs a day—predominately gastrointestinal, analgesic, cardiovascular, and psychoactive. People over sixty-five spend $50 billion annually on prescription drugs, $5 billion of that coming from nursing homes—more than half paid for by the government. A particular nursing home may go bankrupt, but drug use is always on an upward trend. A 2001 survey by the Pharmaceutical Researchers and Manufacturers of America uncovered 261 drugs in development for diseases of aging—Alzheimer's, osteoporosis, and arthritis. This is not to mention drugs for diseases of all ages—122 for heart disease and stroke, 402 for cancer.

Some people wind up in nursing homes only because they can't keep track of their many medications. Is this age related? If you were taking ten drugs a day, how easily could you keep track?

In and out of the rooms the nurse goes dispensing the pills one by one, checking off each on her clipboard. If this were fiction, I'd write that I hear the tune "The Candy Man" coming from one of the rooms.

———————

Finished with Sam, I wander off to approach an eighty-five-year-old woman asleep in her bed. Waking with a start, she screams at me, "Who are you and what are you doing here?"

I am a psychologist who travels around to nursing homes and talks to sad, confused, and, occasionally, happy old people. I work for a company that provides a range of psychiatric services—a team including a psychiatrist, a psychologist, a nurse, and a social worker. Unlike the medical staff that deals in a tangible and ingestible commodity—drugs—I offer an intangible: me. You tell a psychiatrist that the ninety-two-year-old lady in Room 12 is calling out in the middle of the night for her mother, she gets labeled as agitated, and there's a pill that will fix her right up—or so they believe. Sometimes they ask me to change a prescription. "When you guys lowered Mrs. Brown's Risperdal, she became much more delusional." I remind them I'm the psychologist and I only talk to people.

"It's the psychiatrists who do drugs," is my joke.

I get a confused shrug or condescending smile. Then they ignore me.

My eunuch-like quality when it comes to prescribing aside, all of us team members think in terms of disease and cure, in terms of symptoms with an underlying disorder. We're highly medicalized. In order to be paid, we have to come up with a diagnosis. We have a book—*Diagnostic and Statistical Manual of Mental Disorders*—that has a code for everything from anxiety to voyeurism. I look up my diagnosis in the manual and enter the code on a form. I spend as much time writing things down as I do talking to people. No diagnosis, no code, no payment.

But I'm still the invisible man who doesn't do drugs. Not only do they ignore me, they pretend I'm not there. I can be in the middle of Mike Mindykowski's confessing, "I beat my kids. That's why they never visit," when an aide will walk right in and start changing the bed. The maintenance man might saunter in with a mop to clean up the vomit from Mike's roommate. The cable guy might follow the vomit cleanup to fiddle with the TV.

Are you expecting privacy?

In 1996, the Health Insurance Portability and Accountability Act (HIPAA) formalized standards for protecting patient confidentiality. Show up at a doctor's office today and they hand you a HIPAA form outlining your privacy rights. Ever read it? More likely, you're preoccupied with whether that mark on your face is melanoma. You're less likely to pay attention to your privacy rights than the fine print on your monthly credit card bill. It's kind of a joke, actually. All of our medical records and their deep dark secrets are sitting in databases all over cyberspace. Some clerk, possibly in India, seeing you're on Viagra or the date of your miscarriage.

Personally, I proceed on the assumption that the privacy of my own medical records is greatly compromised, and move on from there. For my patients, I do my best. When the aide comes in to change the bed, I jabber about the weather. If there's a roommate in the next bed, I'll do a quick assessment of his mental status. If he's too demented to follow the conversation, I'll assume we're in a zone of privacy. If the roommate is a cogent thinker, I may try to find an empty office or lounge. In nice weather, we might go outside. I may be the first person to remove a resident from her room in days or weeks. With hard of hearing patients, I might close the door so when I shout out, "How's your mood? Are you depressed?" not everyone will hear the answer. If all else fails I may simply draw the Louis XIV curtain around the bed and conduct my session with an illusion of privacy, which doesn't always prevent a roommate from chiming in, "I don't know about her, but I'm very depressed."

This is not psychotherapy in a designer office with leather chairs, objets d'art, and the quiet undertone of a ticking clock. These are field conditions. I'm often moving piled-up clothing or a prosthetic leg to find a place to sit. One of my colleagues abruptly quit after she realized she had been sitting for the past half-hour on a urine-soaked cushion. Sometimes I'll enter a room and then wander off to find a chair to carry back in. I've thought about bringing my portable chair-in-a-bag to be sure of a seat.

The staff's attitude about what I'm doing may be encapsulated in one comment I overheard: "Therapy for these people. What a waste." My patients themselves don't know quite what to make of it. This is the Greatest Generation. Most people in nursing homes are in their eighties, born in the 1920s. Growing up in the Depression, they didn't share my boomer luxury of exorcising their psychic demons in psychotherapy. Food, clothing, shelter, and staying alive were their childhood and youthful priorities, not looking for love and fulfillment in the consultation room. Graduating from grammar school—eighth grade—was a mark of academic distinction. Later they got to escape the farm, factory, or office to be warriors. They're the ones who think you have to be crazy to see a shrink. I don't always specify I'm visiting them for psychotherapy. I low-key it: "I'm a psychologist. Can we chat?" Let them put two and two together however they please. They're often eager for the chat, even if they display an initial reluctance. I have many faults, but in the lives of many of these old folks, I might be the only person who sits down, establishes eye contact, and simply listens.

"How are the kids?" I ask Mrs. Abbot.

I can guess the answer.

"They're fine, but I dearly miss them."

She has a daughter in Paris and a son in Arizona. She can be proud. The girl writes romans à clef for women of a certain age. Her son is an astronomer who spends his nights in the clear mountain air of the Southwest looking for apocalyptic space garbage headed toward earth. There are grandchildren. I see their pictures at various ages, in soccer and basketball uniforms, in high school graduation robes, holding a lacrosse stick at Dartmouth. A much younger Mrs. Abbot, trim and tan, is in one of the pictures with toddler grandchildren at the cottage on Cape Cod. The pictures sit on a French provincial bureau. Above the bureau is a watercolor of a regatta in rough seas.

I could learn to resent and envy her kids, who probably grew up in a home with no yelling, sitting placidly around the dinner table, actually asking, "How was your day, dear?" Bunny—they do have names like that—is the successful writer I dream of becoming, and Junior doesn't have to worry about tuition for his well-mannered kids.

"That's my husband's sloop tacking around the flag well in the lead," she told me proudly, the first time she caught me looking at the watercolor. "I painted it." The painting has the mannered style of someone with skill and time to do it well, but not the drive to be great.

Mrs. Abbot's husband has been gone for more than two decades. She is eighty-three. Charles Abbot II was dead at his Wall Street desk at the age of fifty-seven. He's in the photos too, trim and tan like his wife. I don't envy the heart attack. I'm older than the man in the photo, but alive and reasonably well.

"So how are the kids?" I ask again.

"Bunny is off to Santorini for Christmas, and Junior is observing in the Andes."

The furnishings in this room do not come from Source 1 Medical or Pier 1 Imports. Mrs. Abbot—possible *Mayflower* descendant, Seven Sisters graduate, and daughter of a New England industrialist whose mills have long left New England, first for the South and then Asia—is in one of the upscale nursing homes, Maldon Manor. What you get for your extra money is a building tucked away in leafy greenwood. There are thick—though easy to clean—carpets. You can bring in some of your own furniture. The facility saves a bit on overhead when it's your furniture, and you can get a bit of the homey touch. The staff calls you by your last name—no twentysomethings familiarly addressing people old enough to be their great-grandparents, no "Hi, Annie" to eighty-seven-year-old Mrs. Brown. The halls in Maldon have the required grab railings along the length of the walls but above them are quality art reproductions. A reproduction of Seurat's *A Sunday Afternoon on the Island of La Grande Jatte* is just outside the door.

Mrs. Abbot doesn't get around much anymore. She had a stroke from which she has rehabbed better than expected but not well enough to return home. She can feed herself, and her Yankee accent is only a bit slurred. But she has told me, as I have heard from many others, "If only I could walk."

Feeding yourself is an ADL—an activity of daily living. You get regular ADL ratings on bathing, dressing, getting in or out of bed or a chair, going to the toilet—"toileting" is the term of art for those in the trade—and eating. Your ADL record, a government-mandated requirement, establishes your level of need and care. Mrs. Abbot can feed herself but needs assistance for most everything else.

When her kids make their twice-per-year visits, she gets unhappy knowing that their appearance means that soon it will be months before she sees them again. She's a paradoxical thinker on a level with me who realizes that "Thank God it's Friday" means it's only two days until Monday. Mrs. Abbot stews in her own juices. She used to be a gifted pianist. Last week she didn't leave her room to hear another resident's daughter—a Juilliard graduate—play Chopin on the grand piano in the lounge that exits to the award-winning garden.

"It would have reminded me of all I've lost," she stammers as I sit listening in on her expensive solitude.

Psychotherapy is often weighed down with all kinds of theoretical constructs and elaborate metaphysical superstructures—psychoanalysis, interpersonal theory, client-centered, transactional analysis, cognitive-behavioral. Brings to mind the image in Hesse's *Steppenwolf* of the great composers in hell dragging their orchestrations behind them. But however you frame psychotherapy, it gets down to one person listening to another. Psychotherapy, to have a chance of working, means you talk and I listen—with no agenda except to listen. I work hard to do that. I've had years of training. I've had psychotherapy. It's not easy to learn to listen with no object but to hear what the person is saying. I work hard to check my own *meshugass* (it's a training requirement for shrinks to speak and think in Yiddish) at the door. Freud said that when two people get into bed, other people are crawling in with them. Grace Slick, closet Freudian, sang, "Your mother's ghost stands at your shoulder."

When I sit at a patient's bedside—and bedside manner is all we therapists got—I try to make it just me in the room with her; or not even me, just a mirror that looks like me. I struggle against the feeling that the old lady in the bed complaining her children never visit is a proxy for my dead mother complaining I never visited her. I had a famous professor—Bruno Bettelheim, no less—who told me it's perfectly okay to fall asleep during therapy, just make sure to analyze your dreams. It would be less wear and tear on the soul to be a psychiatrist: simply hand out the pills, free from the collateral damage of a personal emotional reaction.

Annually, according to the Kaiser Family Foundation, we spend $1.5 trillion on health care in the United States. About seven percent—$115 billion—is spent on nursing home care. The $1.5 trillion health care tab dwarfs the piddling $250 billion we spend on cars. In terms of revenue, the nursing home industry ranks well ahead of advertising, publishing, pornography, and the film industry. It's roughly equal to aerospace.

Most people have the naïve assumption that—unlike the rest of the postindustrial world—our health care industry is free market. Health care for the elderly is a mixed economy: private providers largely funded and regulated by the government. Medicare and Medicaid, the two big government insurance programs, pay for most nursing home care. Medicare, government insurance for people over sixty-five, pays for short-term rehabilitation—for example, you are rehabbing a broken hip but they expect you to return home. That accounts for around 12 percent of revenues. But Medicaid—you're in for the long haul and you either start with no assets or have depleted them to qualify—pays for half of the annual $115 billion expenditure. That number represents only the basic costs, room, and board. Billions more in government dollars go into drugs and services such as physical therapists and people like me. And he who pays the piper calls the tune. Because the government pays the bill, it can regulate much of what I do from the minutes I spend with a resident to the forms I fill out to document those minutes.

State governments, typically the public health departments, license nursing homes and psychologists. In Connecticut, I simply ante up $450 each year to renew my license, which expires on my birthday. All I have to do to stay in good standing is to fill out my forms and commit no grievous ethical or legal sins—an undemanding standard.

The homes don't get off as easy as I do. In addition to their licensing fee, they must conform to volumes of regulations, endlessly documenting everything from the movement of a resident to the movement of his bowels, and smile when the state inspectors make their surprise visits. Everyone is on knife's edge—me trying to make my big frame invisible, and the inspectors sweetly asking a nurse why Form 203 is missing in Mr. Harrison's chart. The State can lift your license, rarely, or fine you, less rarely. You can go on the Internet and look up the violations in mom's or dad's home. The ratings are color-coded—like the defunct Homeland Security threat warnings—from green for no violation to red for actual harm or immediate jeopardy. When people from the State are around, they put up a notice on the front door announcing their presence and inviting any family members to come over and chat, which might be a good idea. The State has no statutory requirement to inform you about a problem, even if they discover Mom's diaper hasn't been changed for days.

I get a taste of scrutiny too. All of my notes go on forms that produce a carbonless copy. One copy goes in the chart, the other to my office. Periodically, a Medicare inspector shows up and sifts through my records, making sure I have crossed all the t's and dotted all the i's. Crossing i's and dotting t's could be a violation. Yet the inspector is not a clinician; she's more like a clerk who wouldn't be competent to rate my actual work even if she could read my handwriting.

We all like to complain about the regulations and the intrusive inspections, but it enables all kinds of businesses and professionals to feed at the government trough. A half-century ago, this was a largely unregulated industry. Then came the tabloid shock of snakepit homes—Mom tied to the bed, rats running around, the owner off to jail. The aftermath was the government trying to control not only the quality but also the quantity of services. It mandated an array of services—physical therapy, occupational therapy, nutritionists, speech therapists, activity directors, podiatrists, dentists, and various mental health types.

Outside contractors all, we're not on the staff with salaries and pesky benefits. To the nursing homes, we professionals are free labor. The government pays us. There's a slew of us riding the circuit. I see the podiatrist: "Freddy, haven't seen you since April up at Marston Moor. Heard they went bankrupt."

When a nursing home hires my company or Freddy's, it can advertise it provides psychiatric or podiatric services. When I show up at Mrs. Ickles's door and she asks, "How much is this costing me?" I can say, "It's free. Medicare pays for it." Outsourcing to me is cheaper than hiring staff members with salaries and benefits. When you outsource to Psychiatric Masters of the Universe, Inc., it doesn't cost the facility a dime. All the rest of us are paying for it out of taxes. Who says there's no socialized medicine?

I know people who scoff and call Freddy's podiatry practice and my psych services group nothing but Medicare mills—companies that exist to feed off government entitlements. When the government funds a service, companies open for business will sprout like mushrooms after a storm. But compassion isn't a government mandate, and unfortunately, there aren't enough nuns to go around.

———

Tina Turner sang, "What's love got to do with it?"

Immanuel Kant, the German philosopher about whom a student exclaimed, "I can't understand German no matter what language it's written in!" agreed with Tina. Kant—never married, never in his lifetime more than a few miles from his hometown of Königsberg—said it is not our pleasure but our duty to nurture others. We can't rely on love. It's a dangerous feeling. Feelings are labile. "Tonight the light of love is in your eyes, / But will you love me tomorrow?" Duty is a constant. If a child's welfare depends on its mother's love, what happens when the thrill is gone?

So it was with my father. My care for him was duty fulfilled—regardless of how I felt about him. Thanks to him, I got to experience the other side of the street as a consumer of eldercare services, not just as a provider.

Not so with my mother. In what was arguably a blessing to herself and her family, she up and died in the course of one day. A year before her demise, she survived a serious illness—pneumonia—and maybe her death was an act of kindness in which she recognized the strain her frailty put on her sons, who traveled inconvenient distances to New York City to do what they could.

My parents separated after thirty-seven years of marriage. My emotional landscape contains the residue of two people staying together for the sake of the children. Duty does not always have happy effects on children.

My father is one of the millions who didn't hit pay dirt but did hang on to get to Social Security. He was part of the army of the aged in Century Village, West Palm Beach, Florida—a retirement community for people who don't drive Cadillacs. There was no real estate bubble in this part of West Palm. There were condos that were going for $5,000 in the year 2000, not much more or less than the price thirty years before. Century Village is one of the many places for the elderly that started out with a fresh coat of paint and then aged along with its inhabitants. Many of the residents were lured by its spokesman, Red Buttons, who was a tummler in the Borscht Belt of their youth before he invited them to Florida at the dawn of their old age. Years after they moved to the Village in the 1970s, the ambience looked "lived in." In Dad's apartment, there were rust stains on the bathtub and worn rugs, and the air conditioner breathed as weakly as the residents. Walking around—and you had to watch out for the wide turns the drivers made around corners— it looked like an auto museum of noncollectibles—rusting Fords, Chevys, and Oldsmobiles.

When Century Village opened, most of the folks were in their sixties. They were attracted by the idea of Florida as a place with a golf course, pools, an activity-rich clubhouse, and no snow. Its motto: "We give years to your life and life to your years!" My parents were snowbirds. They drove down to their American dream from Brooklyn each winter for the few short years before it was over for their marriage.

One day, when he was almost seventy, Dad drove down to Florida by himself, leaving Brooklyn, my mother, and a marriage of acrimony behind. Indifference and denial characterized my relationship with my parents. I saw my father about once a year for a few days of stilted, scripted interaction. And so it went for about twenty years, with my denying he was losing whatever grip he had on life.

One day, I made my once-per-week dutiful phone call to Dad and there was no answer. There was no answer through the night and into the next morning. He was a missing person.

My duties to my father—missing or not—were hard to enumerate, being a mélange of biblical, cultural, and family-dynamic injunctions with no clear guidance for the twenty-first century. Throw in my emotional superstructure, and it became even murkier. In my professional life, my government-mandated duties are quite clear. I have a fairly standard routine when I meet someone new. First, I'll do a combined 90801/91600 procedure—psychiatric interview followed by psychological testing. Like everyone else in the medical world, I have codes and procedures, and forms for documentation. I see people who are often not aware that their sons or daughters have signed them up to see me. "Who sent you?" is a common response to my appearance at their threshold. Typically, someone on the staff or a family member will express concerns about a patient—"Mom just sits there all day weeping"—and enter them in the book for referrals. We can't see anybody without a doctor's order, but most physicians are perfectly happy to have us relieve them of the psychiatric burden. They also let the nurses write their orders for them.

My company doesn't make any money on my services. "We just about break even when you see a patient," I was told. The medical people—psychiatrists and nurse practitioners produce a profit. The psychologists are in the mix for merchandising. When my company makes a sales call on a nursing home, our reps say that unlike Brand X Psych Services, which has only psychiatrists, we will provide a full range of professionals, including psychologists. "Full range of services" is a wonderful buzz phrase for marketing.

Bottom line? I'm a loss leader—the cheap gallon of milk that gets you in the supermarket door with the hope that you'll leave with an expensive cut of beef because you have to walk past the meat counter to get to the milk.

Considering how I, a total stranger, am intruding on the privacy of the people I treat, I'm amazed at the responses I get. These people come from a generation not used to spilling their beans to anyone, let alone a total stranger. These are not my fellow baby boomers who enjoyed a pampered search for personal growth—often in a therapist's office. My patients are usually not aware I'm coming, and have no idea why I'm there when I arrive. My usual greeting is, "Hi. I'm a psychologist. My name is Ira Rosofsky, and I'd like to talk with you for a while." Yet despite their suspiciousness, and maybe because I'm the only one who shows them total, undivided attention, they'll tell me their deep, dark secrets.

I start with pleasantries.

"Nice day outside, Mrs. Jones. Where are you from?"

"Brooklyn, New York."

"Oh, really? Me too. I grew up in Borough Park, Ninth Avenue and Forty-seventh Street."

"I'm next door. Bay Ridge, lived there my whole life—until my daughter in Connecticut said it's not safe for me to be on my own. So here I am."

"How do you like it?"

"It's not home."

After the chitchat, it's not long before I'm onto the Beck Geriatric Depression Scale. Mrs. Jones, a private person trying to hang on to her privacy, is suddenly hearing intrusive questions.

"Do you think it's wonderful to be alive?"

"Well, I wouldn't say wonderful. I guess it's better than being dead, but if I woke up dead, I wouldn't be unhappy."

I often get these passive suicidal ideations—PSIs for short. People who would never go and hurt themselves, but wouldn't complain if they "woke up dead," as Mrs. Jones puts it.

There is a fair amount of this comic relief. Two other favorite responses to my stock questions:

"Do you have trouble making up your mind?"

"Maybe."

"Do you have problems with your memory?"

"No, not at all, I have only happy memories."

However pleasant the memories, most of the people I see are unhappy when we meet, but not necessarily clinically depressed. Trading a lifetime of independence for institutional confinement with strangers changing your diapers does not make for happy campers.

After Mrs. Jones spills her unhappy beans, I move on down the hall to the next person. Time is money. I'm fee-for-service, working on commission. I'll spend the required minimum number of minutes per patient, write my notes as fast as I can, get in my car, and get on the road to my next sales stop. I'm a traveling salesman but I carry no products. It's only me.

And it's not always clear who the customer is, the resident or the facility.

I'm sitting in my car after a few hours at Hopton Heath Health Care and Rehabilitation, and my cell phone rings.

"Where are you?"

"I'm just leaving Hopton."

"Could you possibly go back in? There's a problem."

It's wheelchair road rage. The director of nursing tells me that

Tim smashed his wheelchair into Alice. Then Tim and Alice got into a shoving match. Could I please talk to Tim? Could I figure out if it's going to happen again? Is he a danger to himself or others?

I walk over to Tim in his wheelchair.

"How's it going, Tim?"

"Okay."

"Do you remember talking to me earlier today?"

"Uh, no."

"Something happen with Alice?"

"Alice?"

I write down something to the effect that "Tim is as likely to be nonviolent as violent in the future." These weasel words make the director of nursing happy. In fact, she's not at all interested in what I've written and probably won't read it. She cares only that I've documented it—that there's a form with my signature in Tim's chart—which is what she is really concerned about. The State might get a whiff of the incident, and without documentation, it could be a problem or even a fine.

Old age is a majority female terrain. Finally, they're largely rid of us men. According to the Census Bureau, in 2005, sixty-five-year-old men had a life expectancy of sixteen years versus nineteen years for sixty-five-year-old women. Contrary to the notion that longer-lived wives get to enjoy their dead husbands' estates, the data show that old women have fewer material resources than old men do. In 2003, the median income for men over sixty-five was $17,359 versus $13,775 for women. Staying married—if you can manage to keep your husband alive—is the best of all, with a median income of

$36,606. Older single women were almost twice as likely to live in poverty as single men—13 versus 7 percent.

But whatever your gender, if you live long enough, the alternative to death is an ever increasing prospect of disease. Aside from such cheery prospects as heart disease, osteoporosis, arthritis, and stroke, if you reach the age of eighty-five, your chances of dementia are one in two. Before modern medicine and public health, most people died off before they had the opportunity to experience old-age misfortunes. Until quite recently, "Live fast, die young, and leave a good-looking corpse" was the way of all human flesh.

Prehistoric folks had a life expectancy of eighteen. But this brief span was world enough and time for reproduction and survival of the human species. They died too young to have a legal drink, but they had quite enough life span to discover fire and invent the wheel. A handful of twenty-year-old elders was sufficient to pass along a modicum of culture—how to organize the hunting and gathering, how to bury the bodies. Over the next several millennia, as life expectancy crept up to thirty, there was plenty of time to be Alexander the Great, Jesus, or Mozart.

Fast-forward to 1946, the year I was born, and life expectancy was sixty-seven—approaching the biblical three score and ten—quite enough time to invent the computer, triumph over fascism, and replace swing with bebop. People considerately exited before becoming complete demographic undesirables to TV advertisers. You could briefly savor your life achievements in full command of your senses and then leave the scene.

What's the meaning of the extra twenty or thirty years we have attained since my birth? Life remains mortal and finite. Spirituality aside, when you're dead, you're dead forever. There's a scene from a movie—I think it's with Marcello Mastroianni—in which a dinner-party host cuts some flowers but doesn't put them in water.

"Why not put them in water?" asks a guest.

"It only prolongs their agony."

With all the recent longevity gains, how can we say we're not just prolonging the human agony? Thomas Hobbes—who lived more than three hundred years ago, in a time of warfare and upheaval—mused that life is nasty, brutish, and short. Does three centuries of progress mean we can now say that life is still nasty and brutish, yet longer?

The young have a delusion about longevity. They think of the big number but not the frailty, the illness, and the confusion. Ask a typical twenty-year-old, "Would you like to live to a hundred?" and the answer is usually yes, but it's always the Dorian Gray ideal—where you get old but don't age.

Another misconception is that there once was a Golden Age of Family—now lost among our mobile strivers. I always ask the old folks, do you have brothers or sisters? And I often hear, "I have a brother somewhere. I think in Georgia. But I don't know." I get an image of the two of them long ago spending their childhood days at play together, or even sleeping together for years in a shared Depression-era childhood bed. I might see a photo of the two brothers long ago at a forgotten family reunion.

Millions of my grandparents' generation left the old country never again to see their loving kin. Millions of their children left home as young adults looking for work during the Depression— never to return. My in-laws met during World War II in Los Angeles. My mother-in-law was a Finn from iron miners in northern Minnesota looking for war work. Her parents had fled the czar. My father-in-law came from Neapolitans who had migrated to New Haven, Connecticut. He was a sailor on shore leave in Los Angeles. Their grandchildren—my children—have cousins they will never know.

Anthropologists suggest that all Homo sapiens may have evolved from a small band of wanderers, all the issue of a single Eve. All of us billions from a singularity, just like the stars of the universe. And we too are ever flying apart.

Sam's gone too. One day I arrive and someone else is in his room.

"He passed," is the euphemism I hear.

I wish atheist Sam a heaven where he is playing chess with a Russian Communist grand master, or at least no more than a thousand years of purgatory across the board from an unrepentant Trotskyite.

I ask about the new arrival in Sam's room. He doesn't need me. Mr. Jack Mazurkiewicz checked himself in. He's happy to be free of independence and its risks to his frailty.

I have to remember that I'm mostly exposed to the unhappy. Not everyone is a Sam. Jack Mazurkiewicz sits there comfortably, along with his cup of not-too-lukewarm coffee and the Mets on TV. I could think of a worse fate for me.

2 FINDING YOUR WAY HOME

Welcome to the Rest of Your Life

None of my grandparents died in a nursing home. They were all born at home, in the vanished Jewish Ukraine.

I am quite postmodern—whatever that means—yet I am old enough to have grown up in a three-generation immigrant household, where I called my grandmother "Bubbe." She spoke only Yiddish to me and everyone else, and I once was passably fluent in that eternally dying language. My bubbe was the first dead person I saw—one of those early childhood memories. With the coldness of a child's eye, I looked through her bedroom door and saw her lying there. Someone, maybe the doctor on his house call, saw me watching and closed the door on my dead bubbe and my memory.

Some years before I got into this line of work, I would visit Bubbe's daughter, my aunt Fanny, or Faiga, in her nursing home—already a generational change. Fanny was caught between old country and assimilation. From my perspective, she came from a lost and exotic world. To the ultraobservant Hasidim in her Williamsburg, Brooklyn, neighborhood, she was hardly Jewish at all. She made her accommodations, eating kosher but traveling on the bus to visit family on the Sabbath. Her keen sense of justice led her to ridicule what she saw as the corrupt kosher certification racket. "And they call themselves rabbis, taking money to make a *barucha* over the meat." With a smile, she talked of putting some latter-day holier-than-thou in his place.

"I was in this store the other day, and the Hasid behind the counter was ignoring me, as usual. Then I told him I grew up in Latichev and had cousins in nearby Medzhibozh. Then he would have kissed my feet, Ira. But I walked out."

The founder of Hasidism, the Baal Shem Tov, hailed from Medzhibozh and had cousins in Latichev. To reveal that you regularly walked in his footsteps is equivalent to informing certain Catholics that you were one of the child witnesses of the Virgin at Fatima.

Latichev was also the home of Bugsy Siegel's parents and the inventor of the plastic artificial eye, but I doubt my aunt mentioned that.

Aunt Fanny was illiterate in English but had good literary tastes in Yiddish. She appreciated Tolstoy, and had finished *War and Peace*—well before me. From where I sit writing, I can look to the mantel and see a sepia photo of Bubbe and her Russian-born children: Fanny, Bertha, and the baby, Estelle. That photo was taken more than one hundred years ago in our shtetl, where, in November 1943, the Nazis shot all 7,200 Jews—three years before I was born. Fanny, at fourteen, left the Ukraine and traveled with a neighbor family by horse cart and train to embark from Hamburg to Ellis Island, where my grandfather met her. Later, Bubbe journeyed with the rest of the children, including the baby, Morris. My mother, Rebecca, was the love child of my grandparents' New York reunion—the only Yankee, as they liked to say.

I enjoyed chatting with my aunt about literature after I discovered this side of her, which was quite different from the woman who would pinch my cheek so affectionately it would hurt.

"What are you reading, Aunt Fanny?" I asked as I stared at some impenetrable Yiddish title.

"It's Peretz. Short stories. I don't anymore have the patience for anything longer."

I know this Peretz—famous for his mockery of modesty, "Bontche Schweig"—"Bontche the Silent." Bontche is preternaturally humble and pure. He dies, and standing before the Almighty's throne the simpleton asks for nothing more than a hot buttered roll for the morning of every day of eternity. In the background, there's mocking angelic laughter—Oscar Wilde laughing at the death of Little Nell.

"I've been reading Singer—Isaac Bashevis," I replied.

"His brother Israel is okay, but Isaac. Sex, sex, sex. It's a good thing his dead mother didn't have to read it."

In her nineties, she went blind, probably the diabetes, and she's in a nursing home. Times have changed. The old and the frail are no longer hanging on at home with family—a change from my own childhood with Bubbe. My cousins, Fanny's sons, Heschy and Schimmy, are old and frail themselves and in Florida. Fanny stayed on as the Williamsburg of her youth went through its American changes, new immigrants, new cultures, and new foreign languages. My mother would visit regularly on the bus with their sister, Estelle. When I was in town, I'd drive the two of them over to Aunt Fanny's nursing home on Coney Island Avenue—a busy commercial strip. The boxy-looking, nondescript home was jammed between high-rise housing projects, upholsterers, junk shops, and delis of various ethnicities. The blooming buzzing confusion of the home matched the hectic streets in which it was embedded. There was little separation from the street. You opened the front door and there it all was: no lobby, the nursing station to your right, the residents' rooms directly in front of you.

Aunt Fanny proved to me that sound minds do not always live in sound bodies, and they can wind up living in homes that are not home. Aunt Fanny would sit in the hall outside her room while her sisters would fuss and ask around to get a glass of water.

No more Tolstoy for her.

I asked about books on tape. They had them in Yiddish.

"She's not interested," my mom said. "All she says is, '*Genug shoyn!*' Enough already!"

Genug shoyn is Yiddish for passive suicidal ideation.

When I approach a nursing home for the first time, I know what to expect.

The first thing you notice is that there's not much to notice. These are aggressively bottom-line, no-frill institutions. There's no reason to splurge on Frank Gehry or Frank Gehry wannabes. I googled "nursing home architecture" and I found mention of safety, cost-effectiveness, and efficiency—nothing about curb appeal or interior design. These buildings share their design ethos with banks, schools, and prisons. They are institutions that are, well, institutional.

The most likely building will be a one-story affair surrounded by a parking lot—ranch style on steroids. A fraction have a couple of stories. Five stories is probably the Connecticut record.

They are, of course, handicapped accessible. At the entrance, you walk past residents in wheelchairs taking sun and smoking cigarettes and you go through a door that has a big "Open" button if you need to wheel yourself in. In my early days on the job, I could breeze right past the reception desk. But recently—maybe it's 9/11 permeating all—I've had to sign in and out, flash the ID badge clipped to my oxford collar—Ira Rosofsky, Ph.D., over the company logo.

You enter a pleasant lobby—often with leather couches and a chandelier. These are easy touches that impress the public and are unrelated to the level of quality that lies deeper within. I wonder why they bother at all with pleasant design elements. Aesthetic appeal is not in the guidelines of the Joint Commission on Accreditation of Healthcare Organizations. Strictly speaking, you could set up the lobby with plastic lawn furniture—as long as it was safe lawn furniture—and not be in danger of losing accreditation. There is little need to impress prospective residents. Few make a deliberative choice between Home A and Home B. Few plan on a nursing home in advance. Following an accident or sudden illness, most go to the one that has an available bed.

When I assess a resident's mental status, I ask, "Where are we?"

"We're at the hospital?" they often respond.

My patients are often confused, but you don't have to be too addled to conclude that a nursing home is a hospital. The resident likely just came from a hospital and it is hard to see the difference.

Past the lobby, down a corridor, there will be a nursing station with some staff in nursing uniforms and other staff like me in business casual who could be easily confused for doctors.

Accessibility is the leitmotif no matter where you wander. The halls have railings, though I rarely see residents using them. They're mostly shuffling along, pushing their walkers or riding in wheel-chairs. The rooms look like hospital rooms with adjustable beds, call buttons, curtains for privacy, and bathrooms with grab bars.

Accessibility has its limits. Getting in or out of some wards—again the hospital lingo—requires punching a code on a keypad. It's not enough security to deter Jack Bauer, but plenty enough for even the mildly demented.

Aside from the residents' rooms, there are lounges, and rooms for recreation, dining, and therapy. Physical therapy—learning to use a walker after you break your hip, for example—and occupational therapy—learning to feed yourself after a stroke—are mandated services that also bring in revenue, mostly from Medicare (along with Medicaid), the lifeblood of all things nursing home.

Behind the scenes are offices for the staff, institutional-size kitchens, and maybe a staff locker and break room with an array of coin-operated vending machines.

That's pretty much it: lobby, corridors, nursing station, resident rooms, offices, dining area, and physical and occupational therapy.

On any given day there's one or more of a group of circuit-riding outsourced service providers: doctors, podiatrists, dentists, optometrists, and shrink types like me—all mandated by Medicare, all paid for by Medicare or in some instances by its government sibling, Medicaid.

Medicare won't pay for all of us circuit riders. It won't buy you anything from the Wardrobe Wagon: The Special Needs Clothing Store when it sets up shop for a couple of days in the rec room. It won't pay for the hairdresser dyeing your hair little-old-lady blue or the barber clipping your sideburns in the little salon most homes have, complete with drying hoods. It won't pay for that box of choc-

olates you want by the side of your bed—if you're not a geriatric diabetic—and it won't buy any cigarettes for your smoking break.

Medicare will pay only for medically necessary services, which
means it pays for your $200-per-day room and board only when
your stay is part of a rehabilitation program, which can last for no
longer than one hundred days. When your time is up and you're not
going home yet or staying forever, Medicare will continue to pay
for your medical providers, including me, but room and board is on
your own dime. If you can't afford it out-of-pocket or you aren't one
of the few with long-term-care insurance, the other big government
department, Medicaid, will pay for your room and board, but at a
price. Medicaid, not to put a fine point on it, is welfare. To get it,
you have to "spend down"—that is, give up all your assets until you
reach the allowable $2,000 maximum in your banking account, and
then they'll pay the $75,000 per year room-and-board fee for the
rest of your life. Plus they give you $54 each month for wheeling-
around-in-your-wheelchair money, which means you have to budget
carefully between haircuts and cigarettes.

Put this all together, this 24/7 hive of activity, and you wouldn't
need to be more than mildly confused to say to me, "I'm in a hospital." Look at it with a bit more mental acuity and it's a kind of
junior hospital—hospital-lite. It looks more like the hospital in
Young Dr. Kildare—black-and-white, 1938, starring Lew Ayres
and Lionel Barrymore—before the invention of beeping and flashing
high-tech medical equipment. The nursing home is stripped down,
not spaceage. At the nursing station, there's no array of medical
monitors. Maybe there's a board that lights up or buzzes insistently
when a resident pushes a call bell (while I'm thinking, "Will someone go see what he wants already, because the noise is driving me

crazy?"). There's always a chart rack, usually on wheels, for resident records. There's a locked room behind the station for the meds, and there's usually a bathroom I use for my many daily hand-washings at the sink, above which is a detailed seven-step guide to effective hand-washing—a sign that your mother would love.

Most of the residents in nursing homes are accidental tourists. That's exactly how it was for my father.

"I found Dad!"

It's my brother. We've been calling around. His sisters. The neighbors. We're close to calling the police when Robert phones the downstairs neighbor.

"He was taking a walk. He fell and broke his shoulder. I've already called the hospital. He's there for a few days."

It's decision time. Is it time for assisted living or a nursing home? We have a bit of breathing room. Thanks to my dad's service in World War II, the social worker at the hospital says they can easily transfer him to a rehab unit at the local VA. This is early 2000, several years before the VA will overflow with young vets from places like Fallujah, Baghdad, and Kandahar.

No need to rush down to see him. He's in the care of strangers. Every day—I'm even more dutiful now—I call him and hear, "Get me the hell out of here!" Robert and I are thinking it through. Can he stay in Florida or should we ship him up to New Haven, where I live, or Boston, to be near my brother? Independence at home is no longer an option. I'm reluctantly admitting that Dad is losing more than a few miles per hour off his mental status fastball. Prior to this shoulder injury, I was already having problems rationalizing the get-rich-quick schemes of his eighties as innocent replays of the get-rich schemes of his fifties. When I was a kid, our home was littered with gadgets like inkless rubber stamps or the gizmo that repairs windshield cracks—"I just need a contract with a big school-bus company and we'll be set." If you're going to get rich at eighty, it better be quick. Not having a computer, my dad was spared Nigerian e-mails promising a share of $20 million—just give us your bank account log-in so we can deposit your money. But he's sending in money for a scheme that involves buying advertising that no one will read and merchandise that no one will buy. He gets belligerent when I say it's a scam. Fortunately, he can't blow more than his meager Social Security check. But when he blows that and I need to send him money to eat, I cast aside denial.

We could get him into some kind of facility in Florida, but long-distance, remote-control caregiving is a bother, and I don't like the idea of having to travel to Florida—Midwest with palm trees—to keep an eye on things. If it's Boston, that means a six-hour round-trip to visit. If it's New Haven, I could get by managing the situation on possibly only minutes a day.

In New Haven, there's subsidized senior housing where Dad can live in a studio apartment well within the means of his Social Security check. We go for it. Robert flies down to Florida to retrieve Dad. It's one night in the apartment where he spent his last twenty years, and it's off to New Haven. Dad gets a room with a beautiful view of the harbor. We pay for a couple of hours a day of people coming in to clean and dispense his meds. It's not too long before he qualifies for Medicaid, and it pays for the aides and the adult day program. My dad's in day care. My kids are in day care. I'm a card-carrying member of the sandwich generation.

Seeing the depth of his decline, I'm impressed he was able to survive for so long on his own. A few weeks later, he's having only

vague memories of ever having lived in Florida. He still remembers me, but that will change too. With the day program and the
aides, his situation is on autopilot and I feel secure enough to go on
vacation.

A short-lived illusion. Dad falls getting off the bus at the day
program and lands in the hospital with a broken hip. Bad enough.
In the hospital, he crawls out of bed in the middle of the night and
breaks his other hip. The hospital restrains him—his arms strapped
to the bed rails—closing the barn door after the horse has gone. My
brother is hot to sue. My wife, an attorney and a pragmatist, says we
can do what we want but points out that a lawsuit could have limited returns. The hospital might have been negligent, but damages
would not be life-changing. He's not a twenty-five-year-old newly
minted Harvard MBA who got hit in the head by a flowerpot falling off a tenth-story windowsill. What are the lost, future wages
of an eighty-six-year-old demented man? How much more than
zero? Most important, Medicaid would have its hand out for the
lion's share of any compensation. And even if he were able to pocket
millions of dollars, he would still be old, frail, and out of his mind
in a nursing home. This is not to mention the wear and tear on the
soul for my brother and me that would go along with an extended
lawsuit.

After a week, they're ready to discharge Dad to a nursing home.
We don't give it much thought. His day program, which we're content with, is connected to a nursing home. They have a bed available, so that's fine. We think it's temporary, so it doesn't matter where
he is since he'll get home eventually. He never gets home. With two
broken hips and a broken mind, this is it. After we became unhappy
with his nursing home, we put him on the waiting lists for seemingly
better nursing homes. Dad died on the waiting lists. Three years

after he died, I hear from the venerable Mary Wade Home in New Haven—originally founded in 1866 by Eli Whitney's daughter-in-law for "friendless females"—asking me whether we still want him on the waiting list. I tell them the wait will be forever.

You can read all the how-to-choose-a-nursing-home books you want. The reality is, you fall and break your hip and a few days later the hospital social worker is calling around to find an available nursing home bed. Nobody is saying you have to take the available bed, but Medicare won't pay for the hospital after it's no longer medically necessary. They're telling you it's time for rehab at a nursing home, and they will pay for that. My father's story is typical among millions. There is no senior nursing home tour equivalent to the high school junior's college tour. I've rarely noticed a family kicking the tires in a nursing home, wondering if this will be a good place for Mom.

This is not a self-help or how-to book, but I've been in more nursing homes than most people, and as Yogi Berra said, "If you don't know where you're going, chances are you will end up somewhere else." When your dad is in the hospital and the social worker is making noises about finding a nursing home, you might have a day or two to rush around and check them out.

The first Rosofsky rule of checking them out is not to be faked out by the chandelier. It's easy to hang a chandelier in the lobby over the leather couches. But the bottom line for Mom is how long it takes them to clean her bottom. If there are more bottom cleaners per resident in Agincourt Rehabilitation than in Crecy Acres, Mom's bottom will be spiffier sooner, chandelier or not. But finding a home with more bottom cleaners can be a problem. No matter how bright the chandelier, a nursing home has to adhere to only a minimum standard. An astronaut was asked whether he ever got scared on the launchpad waiting for liftoff. He replied, "No more scared than anyone would be sitting on a billion parts all built by the lowest bidder."

Nursing homes operate in a system of quasi-socialized medicine. Everything is pretty much paid for by Medicare (rehab stays of less than one hundred days) and Medicaid (long-term stays after you have impoverished yourself). In the end, the government pays the piper—Mom's bottom cleaner—and calls the tune. In 1987, after loads of bad press—unsanitary conditions, abuse, and neglect—the Feds set national minimum standards for nursing homes. The states, which administer these standards on a local level, can choose to exceed the minimum. As usual, there is a higher level of state funding in, say, Connecticut than Mississippi. But within the states of Mississippi and Connecticut there is a set level of funding per resident and a mandated number of bottom cleaners per resident. So it doesn't really matter whether you're in New Canaan, Connecticut, the richest town in the United States, or twenty miles away in inner-city Bridgeport, one of the poorest, in terms of bottom cleaners per resident. A survey by the Kaiser Foundation concluded that the national median for staff minutes per resident day is two hours, twenty minutes. The Medicaid administration itself says that two hours, forty minutes is the minimum level to avoid serious harm to Mom's bottom. But that is the minimum. The preferred standard is three hours. And for Mom's bottom to be fresh as a baby's, the optimum is four hours per day. No state exceeds the optimal standard. Only two states, California and Delaware, surpass the preferred standard. In Virginia and Alabama, Mom's bottom gets only eight minutes of attention each day.

I remember walking into a beautiful facility—sylvan setting, carpeting, airy public spaces, large rooms—and overhearing the nurses talking about how they didn't have enough staff available for the upcoming shift. "Maybe we can ask Carmela or Anna, if they want to work a double shift." And I remember a scruffy-looking place on a mean city street with dark hallways and small rooms, thinking, "I wouldn't like to wind up here," but changing my mind when I witnessed a superior quality of care.

Nursing homes can be Potemkin villages with pretty façades— leather couches and chandeliers—but with not enough substance to distinguish one from the other where it counts, Mom's bottom. They're all working off the same playbook—the same proportion of staff to residents. So even the Rosofsky rule of not being faked out by the chandelier is largely irrelevant, since the human resources have only to meet the minimum standards.

The art of euphemism supports the façade. I'm not giving you the real names of my nursing homes, so I picked a random state, Minnesota, to illustrate a point about naming. First, you notice that nursing homes aren't called nursing homes. In Minnesota, there is the Bethany Good Samaritan Village, the Golden Living Community, Whispering Pines, and Marshall Manor—names that could easily apply to affluent gated communities. Occasionally, they're health centers, as in the Richfield Health Center. There is the odd establishment that will call itself what it is, a nursing home, but it makes sure to lighten the mood with a name like Pleasant Manor Nursing Home. This reminds me of Century Village. From the street and apartment block names, you would never know this is a mostly Jewish community with a dash of Italians. My father lived on Sheffield. Nearby, there's Elgin, Northampton, Devon, and Kent. A confused Jew or Italian might think he could wander off to the Lake Country for the weekend.

41

I often wonder why they bother with the cosmetic façades and the euphemisms when they're all the same under the skin. All striving for the minimum standard. But ineffably, or maybe it's chaos theory, there seem to be differences. Follow your nose. If it smells bad, it probably is bad. Poop or vomit doesn't smell as bad when it's fresh. Check the nursing station. If you see teetering piles of forms and documents, or if it looks like your teenage daughter's room, the staff is too harried or disorganized to keep up.

I can put in a small brief for religion here. God motivates some of the people to do good work some of the time. Although many religiously founded homes are selling out to corporations, if you see a nun, it might be a good thing. God aside, noblesse oblige among the ladies who lunch also yields good works. The Mary Wade Home, on whose waiting list my father died, evolved from a nineteenth-century charity for "young, homeless girls" to one for their frail elderly great-great-grandchildren. My brother and I liked what we saw—a clean and orderly place, with an apparently active and involved staff. When our tour guide heard Dad was Jewish, she said without condescension, "We don't know much about that religion. We would love to learn more."

We were looking for an exit from Dad's Jewish-run nursing home, which goes to show that religion is not a perfectly reliable guide. That venerable institution, founded in 1914—within my father's life span—is a National Historic Landmark. Dad's day program, also run by his nursing home, was just fine. But even if you're not blind, you can't get a good view of the elephant from one of its parts. When an old family friend, Sid, heard my dad was going there, he said, "My mother was there, a real hellhole!" But he made donations to it—and gave us his tickets to the classy fund-raisers starring Ella Fitzgerald and Joel Grey—so how bad could it be? I told Sid it might no longer be the bad old days.

We found, though, that getting something good to happen was going to be a struggle. The two daily assisted walks—an aide on each arm, Dad hobbling down the hallway—never seemed to happen. Either they didn't have the staff on hand or Dad would command them to "Get the hell out of here!" And they listened to that.

"He says that to everyone," I'd respond.

"We have to respect his rights."

I'd also get the "respect his rights" remark when I asked why he didn't go to the sing-along. Dad liked to sing along.

I'm a rabid supporter of patient rights. But exasperated at his inactivity I would implore them, "He's in a wheelchair. Just wheel him over."

"We can't do that. He has rights."

They were also supposed to walk him over to the bathroom. It was easier for their understaffed selves to put him in diapers. The lesson? If it's easier to leave Dad in diapers, take this path of least resistance—not just at Dad's home, but most places. I, like most parents, find it easier to yell up to my boisterous kid, "Shut up, already!" than to get off my butt and go upstairs and be up close and personal. It was also easier—and assuaged my own guilt—to complain to the staff than to assist Dad on his walks and wheel him over to the sing-along myself. With two elderly parents, three kids, two fish, and a dog, my wife and I are understaffed too.

As understaffed as the staff was, they had the manpower to wage a bitter strike. It's not a good sign when the bottom cleaners risk their meager livelihood to demand more money and better working conditions. During the strike, the administration argued that low wages are a good thing, issuing press releases saying higher wages would downgrade the service.

The philosopher Hannah Arendt looked at ordinary Adolph Eichmann and called the face of evil banal. The nursing home isn't evil. There's no banality of evil. It's simply banal—the banality of banality.

In this highly regulated industry, there's a staffing standard that consumers feel is too low and proprietors feel is too high. There is no incentive to do more than the minimum. In for-profits, the surplus goes into the pockets of the owners. In the shrinking nonprofits, surpluses are theoretically plowed back into the enterprise. This has to be part of the explanation why socialized medicine spends less and gets more.

The United States has the best health care money can buy. But not everyone can afford to buy it. Annually we spend twice as much per capita on health care as Japan, yet the Japanese at eighty-two years are third in life expectancy—just behind Andorra and Macau—and we are forty-fourth at seventy-eight years—behind Bosnia and Herzegovina.

Of course, Japan is a scrupulously homogeneous society. Almost everyone is Japanese. We're an ethnic stew with wide variations in wealth and culture. But Cuba's impoverished status does not prevent it from doing quite a bit better than we do on infant mortality, and only slightly worse on life expectancy. So you don't necessarily get what you pay for. I have a pretty good health care plan, and despite the aggravating paperwork I get the good stuff—the top docs, overkill in diagnostics, payment for expensive cholesterol drugs. About fifteen years ago, I won a negative lottery and was diagnosed with a rare tumor, benign yet problematic—intertwined like a grapevine with the nerves in my left shoulder. I was sent to "the best surgeon in New Haven," and "the best radiologist in New Haven," and "the best rehab doctor in New Haven." But not everyone is so fortunate. Tens of millions have no coverage. They don't even get the worst doctor in New Haven.

Old age's dismal frailty is compounded by Medicaid's requirement that you impoverish yourself before it will pay for your nursing home stay. In Finland, Germany, and Japan, public money pays for you to stay in a nursing home as long as you live, and you can hold on to your assets. We try to game the system by passing on assets to our children—hoping they are Cordelias, not Gonerils or Regans—enough years in advance so that the government won't seize them. If you haven't transferred the deed to your house three years before the nursing home, the government moves in. Most people don't think ahead this way. It's usually the folks who have an estate worthy of estate planning. A Kaiser Family Foundation study found that 7 percent of Medicaid recipients in nursing homes were responsible for two-thirds of asset transfers. And the authors of the study take the hard view that you should give it to the government not your children: "The concern is that the individual's assets should be used to pay privately for nursing home care, instead of being transferred to relatives. Because Medicaid was designed to be a safety net only for the poor, asset transfer practices are thought to distort the intent of the Medicaid program and unnecessarily inflate public spending."

The safety net is only for the poor. If you're middle class, you have to become poor to fall into the net. So much for the American dream of working hard to get ahead.

The bottom line? Because you didn't support socialized medicine when you were young and acquisitive, you could lose everything in order to afford the poorhouse. The moral? Move to Finland.

None of this is to say that the rule of you get what you pay for is inoperative in the culture of eldercare. Consider the end-of-life custody battle in which one-hundred-five-year-old Brooke Astor's free-living, high-spending eighty-two-year-old son lost custody to her grandson. The Astor court documents revealed that negligence is relative. The rich remain different from you and me. Her negligent son provided an in-mansion nursing home room with twenty-four-hour one-on-one care, far exceeding the optimal government standard of four hours.

Even though the Brooke Astor negligent-ingrate-son standard of care remains beyond the means of almost all, the run-of-the-mill affluent can find a place with more care than the two hours, twenty minutes U.S. median.

Salisbury Plains sits at the end of a half-mile driveway off a road that is already in the country. It reminds me of a joke I once heard about Hampshire, a liberal arts college with an affluent student body.

"Why does Hampshire have such a long driveway?"

"To remind the students of home."

As you drive down Salisbury's long and winding driveway, you pass tennis courts and a pool, formal gardens, and stately trees through which you can see the marina on a river that flows into Long Island Sound. The hot summer silence is broken occasionally by the maintenance staff riding mowers across acres of lawns.

This is a retirement community with comfortably large apart-

ments, assisted-living services, and its own in-house nursing home—
the health center, as they like to call it. In the lobby is a photo
of young, vigorous seventysomethings moving in at the opening.
Today, I visit them as frail eighty- and ninetysomethings. The
cohort that came in when the place was new has aged together. I
had a patient, a new arrival at seventy-one, who exclaimed, "I didn't
realize the people would be so old!"

Salisbury Plain is where you go if you are one of life's winners
but not quite on the Brooke Astor level. If you enter the facility
when you are fit and able, you find yourself in a retirement community much like any of the affluent type. You get a nice apartment,
the waterfront, the swimming pools, and linen in the dining room.
If you become a bit confused or a bit frail, they assist your living—
aides can come in and help you get dressed, prepare a meal, or take
you shopping. Nurses come by and dispense your meds. All this for
additional à la carte fees. If you are too frail or confused for this,
you go to the nursing home. It's a pleasant-looking nursing home.
Hushed auditory and visual tones. Carpeting on the floors. No blaring PA system. You still might share a hospital-style room with only
a curtain for privacy. But it's a nice curtain. And your roommate
isn't working class on welfare. He or she is also a former captain of
industry, college professor, or physician.

Philippa Kensington is a ninety-two-year-old Connecticut Yankee who treated me like the help that served her eighty years ago
in Hartford. She is sound of mind but frail of body, sitting in a
Sunrise Wheelchair—the euphemisms extend beyond the naming
of the facilities to the naming of the equipment. The Sunrise lists
for $5,125—well beyond the $900 Medicare will pay for the cheap
Jazzys you see in TV commercials. "You pay nothing. We guarantee

it for free if Medicare won't pay." The top-of-the-line Sunrise—for people whose most recent ride might have been a Lexus—comes standard with "responsive power, smooth acceleration and 'turn on a dime' maneuverability." It tops out at seven miles per hour, faster than most people can run—let alone walk.

"Ira, I have this granddaughter. She's a Philippa too. I love her, but she's a drug addict."

"You must be upset about that."

"I'm beyond upset. I'm very, very angry. I put her through Bennington and it's all going up her nose."

Philippa's dad, Philip, is a warmed-over hippie sculptor who finds objects in the landfill, welds them together, and calls it art. Philip, whose photo shows him in full artist attire—a welding rig and mask in hand, a gray ponytail—is downwardly mobile, no money for Bennington from him.

"So what are you thinking about doing? Can she get help?"

"That's the last help she'll get from me. Either she checks into rehab, which I'll pay for, or it's the end. She can ask her Jew boyfriend for the next check."

I let that slur pass. I maintain my blank-mirror I'm-a-therapist pose.

"Sounds like a plan."

She dismisses me.

"Yes, thank you very much for your help, Ira. I'll call on you again if I need you."

Salisbury Plain is a continuing-care facility. There's a buy-in fee. If you want a one-bedroom apartment, it's $500,000. Less for a studio. More for a two-bedroom. You pay a monthly maintenance fee of $2,500.

There's only one meal per day. There's the belief that old age is an appetite suppressant. Most anyone can pour cereal into a bowl or toast some bread for breakfast in the galley-style Salisbury kitchens. They have refrigerators, microwaves, and toasters, but no dangerous stoves. Many stretch out the one meal for dinner, shuffling or wheeling out of the dining room with lunchtime doggy bags.

Not everyone is happy with the one-size-fits-all menu of assisted-living centers and nursing homes. The other day, a woman sat across from me in her room with a piece of meat loaf the size of a fat hamster.

"Look at this! Who can eat this? And for lunch! I've always had a sandwich for lunch and my big meal at night. Here I can never finish lunch, and the sandwich they give me for dinner always leaves me hungry."

I'm going to have a hard time finding a nursing home that will allow me to sit in my comfortable chair at two a.m., feet up, a whiskey in hand, reading Robert Graves.

I've also learned there's a misconception about assisted living. Ask someone about assisted living, and she will probably say something to the effect of, "Oh that's one of those places that's not a nursing home but where they have people helping you with getting dressed, your medication, and keeping an eye on you."

All true, but for a price.

At Salisbury Plain, the $500,000 buy-in and the $2,500 monthly fee pay for your apartment, the one meal, weekly housecleaning, and use of the facilities. That's about it. Want someone to dispense your meds? There's a fee. Want someone to sit with Momma three hours per day? That will be twenty dollars an hour. Want someone to get Dad up in the morning or into bed at night? The helping hand holds her hand out for another twenty.

So what's all the fuss about assisted living? Can't a body stay in his or her home and pay à la carte for the home health aides, the meal preparation, the getting in and out of bed? That's certainly a possibility—particularly if you're a reclusive type like me. But if you're the sociable sort, assisted living means community. There are people around. There are movies in the auditorium. And there's an emergency staff available twenty-four hours a day if you pull the cord by your bed or in the bathroom. If you don't turn the marker on your door each day, someone will check on you. No need to try your luck reaching for the phone to call 911 like the woman I met who collapsed and lay moaning for days on her bathroom floor, dehydrating, until one of her neighbors wondered, on Monday, how come they hadn't seen her since Saturday.

At continuing-care facilities like Salisbury Plain, there's yet another advantage. Your $500,000 buy-in along with your monthly $2,500 gets you a ticket to the in-house health center, that is, the nursing home. That can be a bit cheaper than the $75,000 it normally takes to live in just any old nursing home. The big up-front payment is a kind of long-term-care insurance. As long as you keep paying the monthly $2,500, it doesn't matter whether you're in your apartment or the more care-intensive nursing home. There's no additional fee. All those $500,000 payments fund the nursing home. This leads to some interesting scenarios. For those with extensive care needs it's cheaper to put them in the nursing home, which is all included, than in the apartment, where you have to pay by the hour for personal care. It also creates some latter-day Jane Austen–type scenarios with the kids worrying about the depletion of their inheritance.

Martin Laurent is one of the world's experts on sonar. He was a physics major concentrating on acoustics when World War II broke out. From Princeton, it was only a short train ride to the War Department in Washington, D.C., where soon, before he graduated, he was in charge of a working group studying the detection of German U-boats. He has told me that despite his many achievements, his parents always made him feel inferior to his younger brother, who became your basic tycoon. It reminded me of the brothers in Joseph Heller's *Good as Gold*. One is a professor and adviser to the president. The other is simply rich. Whom do you think the Jewish immigrant parents favor?

These days, Mr. Laurent sits in his Salisbury apartment with river and forest views. Each week, when I come to see him, he gives me a courtly hello and "Do I know you?" The walls in Laurent's apartment are lined with physics journals, certificates of achievement, and photos in which he appears with two presidents and one CIA director. He claims to give weekend seminars at Princeton, but needs help to make his peanut butter and jelly sandwich on raisin bread. That's when he's not telling his aides to leave. Reminds me of my father, but more polite: "Who are you? Please get out of here!"

His sons are considering this question: How long can Dad stay in his apartment, and when does he need to go to Salisbury nursing home? The unstated question: How long do we continue to cut into our inheritance with the $500 daily payment for around-the-clock aides?

"How do you think my father is doing?" asks Steven Laurent on the phone.

"How do you think your father is doing?"

"Well, he keeps sending the aides away. And some of them have quit. They don't like his racist comments."

"What do you think is best for him?" I ask.

"The agency says they're finding it hard to find aides willing to work with him."

If Dad leaves his apartment and goes to the nursing home, there's no out-of-pocket payment for aides. In the health center, the $2,500 that pays only for the apartment will now pay for room, board, and nurses and aides—and end the twenty dollars an hour for peanut butter on raisin bread.

Several weeks later, I'm at the health center and I see Dr. Laurent. He stares at me quizzically, and I hear, "Do I know you?"

There is a business reason for the posh appeal of the Salisbury nursing home component. Few of its residents came in off the street. When you consider buying a Salisbury apartment, the health center is presented as an important marketing feature. This beautiful nursing home is where you will go if you need to rehab from an illness. Years later, if you need a long-term nursing home, this beautiful place is for you. There's carpeting. The staff calls you by your last name. The furnishings look like they come from Ethan Allen, not Wal-Mart. Step outside, and walk or wheel along the river esplanade. It doesn't matter if I ask you the month and you tell me it's November when it's July: lilacs still in the dooryard bloom.

"We have no Medicaid people here," the head nurse beamed proudly to me on my first visit. "We don't allow them."

Most of the staff—including the head nurse—will probably wind up on welfare when they need a nursing home, but they brag about the affluence of their clientele. Maybe they enjoy the fact that they are diapering their "betters."

Salisbury Plain is where you might go if you were once a doctor, an executive at a Fortune 500 company, a bestselling author, or the spouse of one of the above. This is for life's winners—even if what you have won is merely a nicer version of a shared room with a permanently opened door.

———

I'm talking to Janet Bartoli in the lounge of Bosworth Field. It's on the wrong side of several rivers. Connecticut for all its small size has many regions. The third-smallest state, with 3.5 million people—more than five times the number in the largest state, Alaska—is plenty big enough for regional differences. I know people who live west of the Connecticut River in the Hartford region— Avon, Farmington—who look down their noses at any town east of the river—East Hartford and Manchester. Others joke about inbreeding among the original Yankees in the northeast and northwest parts of the state—our native hillbillies. There's an area in the eastern part of the state that was home to a generation of immigrant Jewish chicken farmers who shunned urbanism to prove that Jews can work as well with their hands as their brains. New Haven, for all its inner-city poverty, remains home to Yale, the Long Wharf Theatre, hot nightclubs, and the Yale Center for British Art, repository of Turners, Constables, and Gainsboroughs. People in New Haven joke about East Haven. The natives and their detractors call it "Staven." East Haven is also the home of big hair, Italian-American style—something I know about from my native Brooklyn. My wife, who grew up there but can't do big hair because of her partly Finnish background, likes to say she was born in New Haven, not mentioning that she left the hospital as an infant not to return until after law school. But the big-hair folks in East Haven still have the locale of the Bosworth Field Health Center to kick around—faded manufacturing towns, tumbledown cottages, and trailer parks. You'll even hear trailer-trash jokes.

At Bosworth Field, the lounge where Janet and I are meeting—

her room too small for a session, stuffed with four beds, clothing piled on chairs—is itself crammed with retired wheelchairs, rickety tables, IV carts, and a TV that plays with a greenish tinge. Janet and I have privacy to the extent that even when Joey wheels himself into the room and parks himself in front of the green TV, he's too disoriented except to ask if I have a light for the cigarette behind his ear. Joey sits there watching *The Price Is Right*, yells "Fix!" at Bob Barker, and wheels himself away.

Janet is on Medicaid, which pays for most of the folks at Bosworth. Janet, blue-collar through and through, aspired to be *petit bourgeois*. She and her husband ran a small contracting company. They had a pickup truck. He worked on small renovation jobs—replacement windows, a deck, a paint job. Janet answered the phone and kept the books. When he died of a heart attack at fifty-seven, the business expired too, and she returned to work as a hairdresser. Later, after she came down with emphysema at sixty-four, Janet's life became too complicated for independence; she wound up in Bosworth shortly after her seventieth birthday.

Janet has no children. Her older sister, Beth, moved down to Florida along with her niece and nephew. Janet hasn't seen any of them for years.

"Beth has that Alzheimer thing. We're both in nursing homes. I don't know how to reach her. Her kids send me a Christmas card every year."

Still sharp, Janet tries to keep busy by helping out around the place as best she can. She's a bingo caller, and could win every week at the trivia contest—"Who was Reagan's vice president?"—if she wasn't kind enough to whisper an answer into the ears of the competition to make someone else's day. The prize is a token, a quarter, and there's nothing to buy.

They referred Janet for suicidal ideation—thinking about death. "I'm not going to hurt myself, but if I die, I don't care."

I write a note she's not a danger to herself or others. In this business, documentation is next to godliness. When the State inspectors come around, they sit for hours at the nursing station going through stacks of resident charts and staff record books. The don't seem to lift their eyes to gaze at their surroundings. The paper is the real thing.

Over the PA system comes the announcement that it's time for the eleven-thirty a.m. smoking break. Janet exits, wheeling her oxygen behind her as she heads out into the February air for two cigarettes.

Bosworth Field is a squat one-story building—cinder blocks with a stucco veneer. The grounds, such as they are, consist of a few benches near the entrance and a concrete courtyard mostly used for the smoking breaks. The lounges are mostly for storage. There is linoleum on the floor, and institutional green on the wall. At the foot of a resident bed is a hand crank to reposition the resident rather than a control panel with buttons. This is the Model T of nursing homes. Patients are often four to a room. Recreation is mostly in one central area, more a widening of the hall than a lounge. Twice a week, evangelicals read the good news of the Bible. On other days, priests celebrate the mass and bring the Eucharist into the rooms of those too infirm or recalcitrant to come to the portable altar. The overall ambience is claustrophobic. In the summer, there is no air-conditioning. Windows are open to the sounds of traffic—unlike the open windows in nursing homes with air-conditioning where many residents are too confused to know to keep them closed.

I have never been to the Soviet Union, and now that it's Russia again, I never will get to go. My wife, a Russian-language major in college, did get to go. Her impression: "The 1950s in shades of drab." This too is Bosworth Field. It's the banality of banality again, the world in black-and-white, before God created color.

Is a scruffy home a bad home? Not always. Beauty in nursing homes as well as in humans is only skin deep. The socially mobile, rootless residents of Salisbury Plain are often cut off from the support of their similarly mobile offspring in faraway places. In the cultural environs of Bosworth there is less mobility; children fall closer to the tree. For some residents, their families are in constant attendance, Louis XIV style, moved by guilt, duty, or love—or all three. Low social mobility means that Mom may get more than four hours of care each day—the nuclear family coming through to meet Medicaid's optimal standard.

Most nursing homes, like everything else in this universe, are somewhere in the middle—neither posh nor scruffy, neither Salisbury Plain nor Bosworth Field, just muddling through like you and me.

Put a Vacancy sign with Free HBO in lights in front of Stirling Bridge Rehabilitation and it could be a motel, maybe two stars in the AAA Tour Guide. It's not Motel 6. It's not the Radisson. Maybe it's the Comfort Inn. It has a mix of welfare residents, private pay people spending down to get on welfare, and Medicare rehab patients. Through the automatic doors, you enter a rotunda off of which are three corridors. To the left is the rehab unit; straight ahead is the long-term unit; and to the right is the locked dementia unit. I don't have much business on the dementia unit. I need a semblance of a conversation to work my magic. My standard for starting psychotherapy with a dementia patient is the possibility they will remember me when I show up next week.

Stirling has neither the peeling paint and linoleum floors of Bosworth nor the artwork on the walls and the patterned carpets of Salisbury. It has institutional carpeting—but carpeting nevertheless—no more than two to a room in which there is always a comfortable chair for visitors, with clothes or a prosthesis to remove only occasionally. In the room, there's room to move around.

Life here is standard issue. You eventually get out of bed; you might go to rehab; you could sit around and watch TV, read, or simply stare into space. There are coffee hours, a men's club, even a Red Hat club for women, along with the ever-present bingo. The Girl Scouts might arrive to do a song and dance. You still might complain about how the staff takes its time to answer your bell, but the bell pleasantly bings, doesn't clang, at the nursing station. And here too there is no jarring PA loudspeaker to spoil your numbing solitude.

This is where I find the woman who lay on her floor for three days before her neighbor thought to inquire.

Agnes Jones, eighty-five, never married. Neither did her dead kid brother, with whom she shared her childhood home for their decades of adulthood. There might be cousins out there somewhere, but Agnes is making her own way in the world. The staff wonders if she is traumatized from her ordeal.

Agnes smiles.

"This is wonderful. The food is better than I ever cooked. I have my TV. And I'm getting around on my walker."

No possibility here at Stirling of three days on her cold bathroom floor. If she falls, it will be on the carpet, and someone will soon walk by.

On the nightstand I see the latest Grisham. Out the picture window, over the hedges, I see the trucks racing by on the highway. But I also see the birds right outside the window, at the feeder.

On a tray, I see the remains of breakfast.

Agnes has achieved her hot buttered roll for the remainder of her eternity.

And there is no mocking laughter from me.

THE RECORDING ANGELS

Doing It by the Book

I t's time for the quarterly care plan meeting at Dad's nursing home. My father, who has a right to be there, is not there. He wouldn't have a clue. I'm sitting at a table squeezed into an office not meant for conferences, fiddling with my cell phone. My brother attends via speakerphone. I chat up a nurse about her golf game. This is the functional equivalent of a parent-teacher conference. We're going over the functional equivalent of a report card.

The golfing nurse—the care plan coordinator—chairs the meeting. Every three months, each of the departments files a report for Dad's chart. Usually the staff moves the agenda along minus the impediment of family, like my brother and me.

First up, the dietitian. But before she begins, we hear an impediment from Robert on the speaker.

"I was in town from Boston last weekend, and there was a banana on my dad's lunch tray."

Dad's kidney has been slowly failing for most of his adult life—slowly enough so something else will likely kill him first.

But bananas and other high-potassium foods are poison. He loves bananas.

"Sorry, I'll look into it," says the dietitian.

I'm personally not at the top of the list when it comes to caregiving time; I'm not spending hours a day or even every week with Dad, but I worry about the bad kidneys of residents whose families never show up.

The doctor never attends care planning. A nurse drones on about Dad's vital signs and the ups and downs of his meds. There's no physical therapist, either. My dad has "plateaued." There is no hope of additional progress for his fractured hips. Medicare won't pay for plateaus. Exercise would still be good for his hips, but he'll have to get someone other than Medicare to pay for him to walk across a plateau. Pushing ninety, he's a Medicare orphan. My brother and I pester the recreational therapist and the social worker about exercise, having the aides walk him. This is when we get the lines about staffing shortages, and how he doesn't want to go on walks, anyway. Neither does he want to go to recreation.

"Forget about his rights and just wheel him down to the damn sing-along!" I implore.

They write that down.

Three months later, we'll do it again.

Everything is written. *Maktub* in Arabic.

You may think you're in something like a home, but you're a 24/7 patient for the rest of your life. It is written. *Maktub.*

When I show up at a nursing home, I obsequiously ask for leave to plant my butt on a seemingly unoccupied nursing station chair. If

I pick the wrong seat, I'll hear it. "You can't sit there." The nurses won't say that to a doctor—although they might to one of our consulting psychiatrists—but I'm not a real doctor, anyway.

Approached from the outside, the station appears as a rampart. The staff walled off from the outside world not quite bank teller style, but if you're in a wheelchair, you're pretty much like the child who can't see over the candy store counter. Sometimes residents wheel or walk in and plant themselves and maybe idly pick over some papers. The staff might tolerate this or even distract the resident with a stack of blank paper to play with. Often they wheel them out and the resident continues on his wanderings. Occasionally, there's a door and a latch at the station's entrance that is beyond the competence of most residents.

If I do find a place to sit, and I'm alone writing my notes, an ambulance driver pushing a gurney will ask me which room for Mr. Hivers. A drug deliverer asks for a signature. A resident asks for his cigarettes, another for her mother. I get off with, "I don't really work here."

Behind every nursing station is an inner sanctum I never enter. Only a nurse can hold the key to the med room—the donjon, the keep.

My business, my only business at the station aside from schmoozing when I'm in the mood, is the charts. Drugs are passed out once every eight hours—like Jewish prayer, three times a day. The charts on their racks are always with us—ordinary unsanctified life. Rows of fat loose-leaf binders, swollen with paper and divided into many parts. I googled "nursing home chart parts," and the first hit is Nursing Home Advocates. Initially, I'm thinking it's a political action group, but it's lawyers "FOCUSED ON NURSING HOME NEGLECT AND ABUSE LITIGATION"—in capital letters, no less. They advise potential litigants to "periodically (every month or two) ask for copies of these records to make sure they accurately reflect your observations and the care provided to your loved one. In making your request, advise the staff that you are the eyes and ears of the family and you want to be in a position to provide the staff with accurate and detailed information."

As my daughter would say, "As if."

I know of no eye or ear of any family that has joined the chart-reading club. I'm a high poobah of the club, but I didn't bother with my father's chart. I could predict the contents. I attended the care planning and knew what I would find. In my private life, I didn't sit for hours reading about my tumor. I have an elderly neighbor who didn't open the letter we had all received about the big rise in property taxes.

"I knew it was bad news, so I just put it in the drawer."

I can relate.

But I have no problem looking into the records of other people's lives. There's emotional distance. It's a duty.

On the binding of a chart is name, room number, and doctor. The information is temporary, written on a card that slides into a clear plastic slot, as are the room numbers and doctor. Discharge or death, and you slide out the ID card, send the guts of the chart down to the archives in the basement, and recycle the binder with a new resident's records.

If the resident is off to the hospital, they flip the chart on its side in the rack, meaning there's hope for a return, but no guarantee.

When I open an active chart, there's the face sheet. If the chart were a book, the face sheet would be the title page. There's the name and address, family contacts, and social security number, a field of dreams for an identity thief. I always check the birth date with interest, like a coin collector sifting through the ordinary Lincolns for a wheat straw, looking for the rare find of a birth date like 1906. Everyone wants to be one hundred; today I'll get to meet that person. And there's the odd amusement of a note in bold print from Bob Salmon's conservator forbidding his ne'er-do-well son from ever visiting. Dad was not happy when Junior cleared out the joint bank account to buy himself a Corvette, leaving him with only a wheelchair for wheels. But mostly I'm interested in getting the name right and the insurance ID number so I can be paid for my face time with Mr. Salmon.

The next section might be consents. Consents to see me. Consents to have the facility store some valuables. A consent to let Mr. Salmon die instead of being resuscitated.

There's a section for physician orders. Docs don't ask "please"; they issue orders. Because I'm often confused for a physician, as I'm leaving, a nurse might ask, "Did you leave any orders?" I tell them no, that I'm only doing psychotherapy and psych testing, and I get the puzzled "Oh." The docs issue orders for drugs, orders for consultations, orders that Mr. Salmon be rotated in bed every thirty minutes.

There's an Admissions section—as they say in the literary trade, the backstory. I see how Mr. Salmon caught pneumonia and went to the hospital. Then he was too sick to go home but well enough for the nursing home.

Next are the Progress Notes, mostly by the nursing staff, about how Mr. Salmon ran a fever last week but went to bingo yesterday. And there's a section for the mandatory physical exam—a time when the physician is actually hands-on with the resident—that is, unless he sends his physician's assistant to do the job. Most of the medical practice is remote-controlled by the invisible, often absent, hand of a doctor's order. You think this isn't a job that could be outsourced, but considering how little time the docs spend with the residents, I can imagine Dr. Bujhindar on the phone from New Delhi not from New Haven.

Each department that paraded before me at my dad's care planning meeting—physical therapy, occupational therapy, dietary, recreation, psychiatry, and social service—has a chart part with notes, orders, and evaluations.

Nursing has a big section, documenting minutiae such as vital signs, wound care, bed turnings, and excretory function. You crash into your neighbor with your wheelchair, they write it down.

Summing it all up is the minimum data set (MDS)—an omnibus report card. In mind-numbing detail, the MDS includes resident demographics; customary routine cognitive patterns; communication, hearing, and vision patterns; psychosocial well-being; physical functioning and structural problems; continence; disease diagnoses and health conditions; oral, dental, and nutritional status; skin condition; activity pursuit patterns; medications; special treatments and procedures; discharge potential; and influenza and pneumococcal vaccine immunization status. The MDS is required for all facilities that accept Medicare or Medicaid. Each nursing home has a paper-pushing RN—the MDS coordinator—whose job it is to compile the data and pass it on to the State. The State compiles these compilations and passes them on to the Feds for yet another compilation. The recording angels keeping tabs on you.

Multilayered tabs. The MDS is constructed out of resident assessment protocols, RAPs, which are not to be confused with activities of daily living, ADLs, which themselves become part of the MDS. The ADLs answer some of these questions: Can you do a full-fledged bath or shower or at least bathe yourself with a sponge? Are you able to use the toilet or do you need diapers? Can you get up and walk or at least transfer from bed to chair? Can you feed yourself or do you need someone to feed you?

As Rabbi Shila said about the work of the recording angel, "All his deeds are enumerated, with place and date of occurrence." As I said, "There is one book that tells the nurse what to do, and there is another book where she writes down that she has done it." It reminds me of my brother's college roommate, who, if he went to the store, would write down in a little book, "3:33 p.m. Drove to 7-Eleven and back—2.4 miles." I don't know if he recorded his bowel movements, but he would have made a perfect MDS nurse. He did become one of the world's foremost experts on railroad scheduling.

Aside from the charts, there is a groaning board of other documentation, typically in loose-leaf binders, at the nursing station. My company contributes to this with our communication book, in which the staff makes referrals, in which each of us maintains a list of our sessions with residents, and in which we talk among ourselves about what piece of business is to be done next. At any nursing station there are sagging shelves bearing a variety of tomes other than the resident charts. I was at one station searching for our referral book and stopped to marvel at the books and binders lined up on a long shelf. In no particular order, here's what I found: Nursing Care Plans, Wound Care, Primary Policy Procedures, Cart 1 Flowsheets, Cart 2 Flowsheets, Visitors, Communion Records, Exposure Control Plans, BM Record, Nursing Communications for DNS, Volunteer Sign-in Book, CNA Sign-in book, CNA Sign-out book, MMH Drug Log, Body Audit Log, Staff/Resident Activity Involvement Log, Drug Disposal Log, Resident Activities Log, CNA Communication Log, CNA Error Log, Tube Feeding Chart, Weight Book, W-10 Emergency, Housekeeping Notes, and Transportation Book.

And now the punch line: I found a copy of *The Paperless Solutions User's Guide.* "It's time to eliminate your paper files!" As if.

Who reads this BS?

The State shows up for its unannounced inspections. I see the note posted on the front door alerting all who enter that the State is around to promote quality of care. I tread lightly, and so does everyone else. When the State's around, I don't ever read a chart sitting in the corridor on a spare wheelchair next to a babbling octogenarian. It's the nursing station for me. I might even introduce myself not as Ira. "Good morning. I'm Dr. Rosofsky."

In addition to sniffing around the physical premises and asking questions of staff, residents, and families, the State will pull some random charts and read right alongside me. First, they check for all the required parts. Next, they drill down a little deeper, looking to see that each note has all its required parts and that the notes are signed and dated. And I know the State looks for red flags, such as my note about a resident throwing his paper cup with no follow-up incident report.

If they don't like what they see in the chart or in the building, they can issue a fine or harsher sanctions, such as probation or— very rarely—the death penalty: loss of license.

My forms are designed mainly to accommodate governmental requirements. In *Amadeus*, Mozart protests to the emperor that his music has exactly the notes it needs—no more, no less. Our forms are designed to have exactly what the State needs—no more, no less. At one staff meeting, the main topic was how we were losing reimbursement because some of us were forgetting to check some boxes and fill out every line. "Please, please, remember to file a complete form." The meeting didn't have much talk about clinical practice, only about check marks. This is a business, people. Be efficient. Be productive.

Periodically, with the government visit in mind, my company prescreens my forms and lets me know I forgot a signature here, a date there. Rarely the question: "How's the therapy for Mr. Salmon going?"

But the State doesn't poke around every day, so is anyone reading the charts when they're not checking for check marks?

Doctors or their minions might read the charts to remind themselves which meds and what dosage they recently prescribed. I look at the charts to get some background. Widow or widower? Children? Do they visit? Medical conditions? Are they terminal? Age? Date of admission? Meds? I always check the insurance coverage. If you don't have Medicare, then it's sorry, wrong number. In our balkanized medical insurance system, Medicare will always pay me, but if the insurance is managed care, then we'll need preapproval, which, approved or not, means unreimbursed time hassling with clerks and their bureaucracies.

So the staff, the residents, and I are living life by the book. Endless carpal tunnel writing. Spontaneity is suspect. Do something unpredictable and they write it down. Spontaneity is processed and comes off the assembly line as a progress note. Progress toward what? If a patient asks, "Are you writing this down?" I might note, "Resident asks if I'm writing this down." We're getting the experience we need to work for the FBI, opening files on citizens who call and ask if they have a file.

This busywork is not unobserved.

Arrayed around the nursing station is a group of residents lined up in wheelchairs. The barbarians at the ramparts? Or the easiest way for the staff to keep an eye on troublesome patients—the ones who will try to stand up and walk away, or stand up and keel over? I hear the beeping and buzzing and ringing of unanswered call bells at the station, and I hear these siren alarms—WanderGuard is one brand name—going off when butts leave wheelchairs. I hear choruses of "Don't stand up, Mr. Salmon!" Salmon will sit down. They think he's redirectable. But a few moments later, he stands up again, echoing the sound of sirens.

I, too, set off alarms. I sit on an alarmed bed. If I squirm just right, the siren sounds and Mrs. Hayes in a wheelchair beside her bed might stare blankly at me and ask, "What's that sound?" Sometimes I can figure out how to disarm it. Other times, I'm chasing after an aide, "Could you please help me here?" I don't know if it makes her day to see what an idiot a doctor can be.

Stanley Technologies, the folks who brought us garage-door openers, manufactures WanderGuard. Stanley is both revered and reviled in Connecticut, particularly in New Britain, where it started in 1843 and brought fame to the town that became known as the Hardware Capital of the World. Joan Crawford would shut down this birthplace of the wire hanger. But no need. Stanley seduced but later abandoned New Britain. Many of the residents worked in their youth for Stanley and its manufacturing brethren. The jobs went south before going to Asia. Despite its Anglo name—New Britain—this is no home of the apocryphal Connecticut Yankee. It's also nicknamed Little Poland. In 1969, before he became Pope John Paul II, a Polish cardinal, Karol Wojtyla, celebrated mass at Sacred Heart Church.

Stanley tried and failed to reincorporate in an offshore tax haven, Bermuda, but did manage to lay off thousands when it could not compete with cheap third world tools. It transformed itself into a service company and the reseller of electronic gadgets like the Wander-Guard, which are manufactured somewhere else. The butts of the last generation of workers who could feed their families on the Stanley payroll are now kept in their wheelchairs by WanderGuard: "Portable in design and flexible in function—monitor patients who are undergoing rehabilitation, who suffer from a head injury or dementia, and/or geriatric patients who represent a flight risk or exhibit aggressive behaviors."

The truly recalcitrant—those who will stand up forever and again—are physically tied to chairs and beds. Of course, they ask for consent from the family, but what choice do you have? After my father climbed out of his hospital bed and broke his second hip, they tied him to his bed rails with straps around his wrists even though he had no third hip to break.

But only the incorrigibly recalcitrant are tied down. As late as the 1950s, psychiatric hospitals, as well as nursing homes, widely employed physical restraints. These were not the sore-inducing iron chains of Bedlam but soft leather straps, straitjackets, and padded rooms. Then a French surgeon, Henri Laborit, tried a heavy-duty tranquilizer called chlorpromazine on some apprehensive pre-op patients. They became so drugged out that they felt little pain and needed less anesthesia. Laborit thought this could be a boon for psychiatric patients too, but he encountered resistance from a field then relying on electroshock therapy, lobotomy, psychoanalysis, and physical restraint. Eventually a struggling pharmaceutical company, SmithKline, bought the American rights to the drug. They renamed it Thorazine and marketed it to state hospitals as a patient-care cost saver. Tranquilize your crazies and lay off some of the big, beefy orderlies. And so dawned the chemical restraint revolution.

But dementia is a powerful force against reason or restraint, possibly more powerful than psychosis. My dad on Depakote—a descendant of Thorazine—still had to be strapped into his bed at the hospital, and when he went into his nursing home, he was held in his wheelchair with a seat belt—with my permission, or course. The rights of patients meant that my father might not be wheeled off to the sing-along against his irrational will, but a stroke of my power of attorney signature was sufficient to restrain him.

They up the ante for those more clever than my dad—those who can unhook the wheelchair's seat belt. They escalate to a tray that attaches to the wheelchair's arms. Imagine being permanently stuck in your seat by an airplane food tray, and you get the idea. I can be sitting at the nursing station minding my own business, writing my notes, when a resident will roll by and ask, "Can you get this off me?" I'll smile, say "No," and he'll roll down the hall asking us all, "Can you get this off me?"

I see all the contraptions roll by, my eyes wide open at the cage with wheels that surrounds the human as he walks his way around the halls. It has a seat when you're tired of walking in your portable cell. But don't call them rolling cages, they're Merry Walkers.

Given that chemical and physical restraints are not foolproof, the staff takes additional measures with its more recalcitrant charges.

That's one of the reasons for the array of wheelchair residents lined up in front of the nursing station. These residents spend the day watching the staff watch them. The more lucid, or at least the more verbal, or those who can make any sound at all, are a Greek chorus that comments on everything and everyone. "There goes a big one," I hear as I wander by.

Not all the chorus is verbal. There's the Scream Lady. She sits silently in a wheelchair, her face frozen permanently in the shape of the eponymous figure in the Edvard Munch painting. In my imperfect memory, I swear I recall silent tears running down her face every day at one p.m.—her scream face a permanent mask, much like those worn in the ancient Greek chorus.

This is where I find Mr. Ackroyd and his incessant "Help! Please help!"

And there's my dad. He's in the chorus too. They tell me he's not safe in his room alone. He greets me with his customary "Get the hell out of here!" But he doesn't know who I am as he accepts the chocolate-chip cookie from my fortunately oblivious-to-insult three-year-old son.

Behind the station, all of us busy bees are sitting with the charts, pens out, occasionally staring at the chorus before us. I don't know how much reading is going on, but I'm sure about the time going into the writing. I look for the fattest pens for my stubby fingers, so they won't ache at the end of the day. My time is divided into two parts: visiting with residents and writing about them—the writing taking almost as much time as the visiting.

Reminds me of an early supervisor who said at a staff meeting, "I think we should just lock all the offices, so the professional staff would have to spend their time in the day room with the patients." They fired him a few days later. Maybe it was that statement. Maybe it was because of his belief in astral projection, but I'll steal his idea and call it the Rosofsky Law of Inverse Proportionality: The more training you have, the less time you spend with patients.

The rationale for this, I suppose, is the belief that a highly trained expert's knowledge, wisdom, and expertise will diffuse itself—dare I say, trickle down?—to where it's most needed. If an M.D. or a Ph.D. spent all his time with patients, his wisdom would be lost on the less experienced, the less well-trained staff. But is this any more than the psychiatrist saying, "My time is too valuable for actually seeing patients?"

The irony is that the least-trained staff—the aides and the housekeepers—spend the most time with the residents. They are more likely to come from the same economic and cultural strata as many of the residents. These salt-of-the-earth staff are more likely to stop and chat unpretentiously—their talk unfiltered by pretension or training.

There is a study, possibly apocryphal, that pitted grandmotherly *yenta* types against highly trained psychotherapists. The therapists did their polished thing, and the grandmas did their yenta thing. In this non-double-blind study the grandmas did just fine. No one has studied the effectiveness of CNAs as psychotherapists, but I imagine they would do as well as apocryphal grandmas.

But whether they are doing as well as me or other professional staff, their extensive face time with residents is a fact of nursing home life.

Three times a day at the nursing homes, there's a shift change— seven a.m., three p.m., and eleven p.m. I've never been there for the eleven p.m., when I'm normally within the bosom of my family. And I've never been there for the seven a.m. Given my own Oblomovian tendencies, if I'm awake at that hour, I am probably getting the kids ready for school. The early bird gets the worm, but who wants a worm? I've learned that for the likes of me, it doesn't pay to arrive too early at a nursing home. I initially tried to show up at nine a.m., but most of the folks were still in bed. Even when I arrive at ten, it's hit-or-miss whether they will be ready to talk to me.

I have been at the scene of many three p.m. shift changes. It's a time when I am careful where I sit and don't bother anybody. Around the nursing station is a gaggle of CNAs obscuring the wheelchair Greek chorus.

First they hear the report.

"Mr. Jones. He's fine."

"Mrs. Alabaster. She threw up and is running a fever. Keep an eye on her. We may need to send her to the ER."

"Mr. Robb. He tried to choke Mr. Forsyte. Keep an eye on him. I'll be sitting here writing up the incident report."

"Mrs. Leeds. She said, 'If I had a gun, I'd shoot myself.' We'll put her on fifteen-minute checks."

Mrs. Leeds had a stroke and couldn't hold a gun even if I handed one to her. But suicidal threats get attention. If someone committed suicide, that would be the mother of all incidence reports. I've never seen it happen, but I've seen the police show up after a resident-on-resident assault. At one nursing home, there was an arrest and a scandal after a middle-aged, relatively able resident sexually assaulted an eighty-year-old woman.

After report, the nurse divvies up the assignments. On the grave-yard shift—they say "graveyard" only with the sincerest blackness of humor—when the residents are mostly asleep, you can get away with only a skeleton crew (more black humor). During the day, when they're getting up, getting out of bed, going to activities, getting poked, prodded, and getting back into bed, you need more staff. I've seen as many as one CNA per five residents, and as few as one per twenty. I've already outlined how the care in minutes per resident ranges from abysmal to below standard. Another government study indicates that the average care per resident per shift was sixty-four minutes. That includes all staff—CNAs, nurses, therapists, and possibly me. On the classic Ford assembly line, you might have five seconds to turn your screw as each car passes your station. But at the end of the day, you could look at all the cars rolling off the line. In nursing homes, there is no product at the end of the day. No car you can point to and say, "I made that." I know of no nursing home that acknowledges this irony with a name like Sisyphus Health Care and Rehabilitation.

Martin Buber foresaw this in 1923 when he wrote *I and Thou*. I doubt he was thinking of nursing home residents when he wrote we can relate to others either as "I and It," or "I and Thou"—similar to Kant, who spoke of treating others as ends, not means. "I–Thou" comes down to the simple idea of encountering other humans authentically without preconditions—subject to subject—the way we might encounter God. "I–It" is objectification.

Not that "I–It" is always a bad thing. When I was in the midst of my medical adventures with the rare tumor—surgery, painful exotic radiation procedures, and several bouts of general anesthesia—I found it quite useful to objectify myself. I was not a human, a person. I was an object being acted upon. I could weep and moan and bitch on the dawn of eight hours of surgery, but whatever I did, however I felt, in eight hours it would be over. Better to think of myself as an object being processed through the procedure, a car on an assembly line, a resident in a nursing home. The scalpel was entering me not as "I" but as "It."

Seneca, the Roman philosopher, who accepted the Emperor Nero's invitation to kill himself, wrote, "Fate leads the willing, and drags the unwilling." Life is a dog tied to a cart pulled by a horse. The dog has the choice to follow willingly or to be dragged wherever the cart and horse go. This worldview redounds through the ages. The Alcoholics Anonymous serenity prayer—an adaptation of a prayer by the theologian Reinhold Niebuhr—is pure Stoicism. "God grant us the serenity to accept the things we cannot change, courage to change the things we can, and wisdom to know the difference." Maybe you didn't know Mother Goose was a Stoic, too:

For every ailment under the sun
There is a remedy, or there is none;

If there be one, try to find it;
If there be none, never mind it.

Stoicism was a perfect fit for the Roman Empire, reassuring emperors of their position and enjoining slaves to know their place. Marcus Aurelius, an emperor, and Epictetus, a slave, were two of its luminaries. It's a good fit for any hierarchical society. There may be pie in the sky when you die, but not in this life. But it does have its uses. It's a consoling philosophy. On my way to the operating room, I chose to be the dog who walks right alongside the cart—or, to be precise, actually rides on the gurney—rather than the dog who gets dragged to anesthesia and the knife.

And that's the way it is in the nursing home, as well as any other custodial institution whose purpose is to get a body from the beginning of one shift to its end. The staff treats you like you're tied to the cart, and they want you to go where they take you. You might get a little empathy, but it's not in the job description. Like my own bloodless Kantian duty toward my father, the staff has duties but hugs are not required. A little bit of "I–Thou" wouldn't hurt, but it's hardly necessary.

Which brings us to the Hoyer lift. In this objectifying, industrial environment, there is a fair amount of specialized, industrial equipment. Much of the equipment feeds the record-keeping machine: electronic thermometers, scales with chairs for those who cannot stand, muscle testers, inclinometers to measure the tilt of a head or a spine. There's an assortment of walkers, wheelchairs, canes, and crutches. The beds have push buttons or cranks. The food arrives in aluminum cabinets with shelves—to keep it as lukewarm as possible. The medicine moves down the corridors on wheeled carts. Flipping through the pages of a nursing home supply catalogue—seeing shoulder-mounted hair rinse trays and folding canes—my reaction is, "What will they think of next?"—illustrating the ingenuity of human invention reaching into its most obscure parts.

The Hoyer lift is a device for lifting people that minimizes human error and the human touch. Take a construction crane that lifts steel girders, shrink it down to human scale, and you have the Hoyer lift. There's a wheeled base, supporting a vertical rod, from which two insectlike arms suspend a sling. Insert human into sling, turn the crank or, on power models, push the button, and the hydraulic mechanism lifts you out of bed into your wheelchair. Only two CNAs are required.

This is usually done in private—that is, with the curtain drawn. But sometimes they forget to draw the curtain and I see a resident swaying in the air while aides wait to see who wins Showcase Showdown on *The Price Is Right* at eleven forty-five a.m.

Time was when a resident had to get out of bed, several aides would gather around and lift him pallbearer style. It was a hands-on human touch experience. I'm not saying that there was a golden age of nursing homes. In the unregulated past, there were probably more bedsores, infections, uncaring neglect, and deliberate abuse. All the regulations about which I complain do some good, save some lives, and get the residents to the next shift without obvious signs of abuse or neglect.

An industrialized, objectified existence, handing you off like a relay-race baton to the next shift. For all its abuses, though, the old way was a hands-on, labor-intensive experience.

I'm sitting with ninety-one-year-old Mrs. Mullaney in her room overlooking Connecticut woods.

"I'm very mad at that man of mine."

"Mad?"

"For leaving me."

"How long ago was that?"

"He died on me six years ago, and here I am."

The psychiatrist called her demented, but I look it up and she's accurate about the six years of widowhood. She tells me, "I don't have long to wait before I see him." But now she's waiting for bingo in fifteen minutes, sitting at the door waiting to be wheeled down.

Maybe, in her case, I can use the intensive, obsessive record-keeping to do her a bit of good and save her from the dementia label, and from living in the dementia ward—noting and underlining that she knows the date, the town, and all the details of her sad abandonment by that man of hers who dared to die. Beyond only writing a note, I walk over and tell the nurse out loud that Mrs. Mullaney is definitely not demented. Everything is written, but not everything is read.

We'll see if it helps. Even if she stays out of the dementia ward, it won't much help her outlook on the future.

I don't want to spoil your reading pleasure, but I'll give away this book's ending: Everyone dies. When you can't go home and are permanently in the nursing home, they ironically call it long-term care. Most long-term-care residents last two or three years. Long-term care means you are on the banks of the River Styx waiting for the ferryman, or maybe you're already on the ferry. At least that's what's on the mind of those who still have one.

"I'm ready to go," says Mrs. Mullaney.

"To bingo?"

"No, to die and yell at my husband for leaving me."

It's not just the staff who's going through the motions.

OLD AS A STEINWAY

Cast of Characters

Driving home one day, I took the scenic route—a mostly straight-line two-lane blacktop, punctuated by some of Connecticut's few rotaries, bracketed by the occasional but tastefully appointed strip mall. Nearing home, I noticed a piano store. We already had a piano, a workaday upright, Linda's childhood companion. I don't play piano or anything, but we had embarked on a search for her childhood dream, a grand piano, and had been dipping our toes in the treacherous waters of finding just the right one. Walking past the plebeian Knabes, Chickerings, and Baldwins, I noticed an aristocrat, a Steinway—perfect but for the "Sold" sign.

"Too bad it's sold," I said.

"Well, actually it's on deposit, but they're not sure they're going to take it."

"Is there a problem?"

"Not with the piano. They're worried it might be too big. If you're interested, give me your number, and if they change their minds, I'll give you a call."

Too big? It was a measly five feet, eight inches long, a hair taller than Linda herself, who is not short for a woman, but maybe for a piano. She had painstakingly indoctrinated me about piano size. It would have to be significantly taller than she was. My six-foot, three-inch height would be a good starting point. The Victorian design ethic is: Too much is not enough. And when it comes to a grand for the Victorian house that Linda lives in, too big would not be big enough. Size matters.

There is no grand that's too grand.

I'd look at our small sitting room and she'd say, "I see no problem with seven or even eight feet," as I'd imagine crashing into a massive concert grand while groping my way to the bathroom in the dark. We had a paper cutout of various piano sizes, and she'd lay them out on the floor. "Look, even nine feet fits right in."

I remained dubious but figured a grand piano could be a cheaper way through a midlife crisis than a BMW. A run-of-the-mill middle-class family like mine can aspire to have the best piano.

Everything falls into place for Linda. The next morning. she rushes over to play it. What's not to like? Our piano tuner calls it a "gem." The people who left a deposit foolishly decide it's too much for them. And even though we can afford it, Linda's mother, Helen, offers to pay for it—an offer we didn't refuse.

Linda quite happily settled for the five-eight Steinway, rather than, say, a six- or seven-foot Yamaha. A Steinway is a Steinway, even if it is a Model M—a model deliberately downsized from the Model L, made smaller for the apartment-dwelling urban population of the 1920s, a few years before they would give up pianos for radios.

None of us missed the irony that Linda's mother was as old as the Steinway—both born in 1923. The Steinway was put together in Queens, New York, in the Astoria factory. Helen saw the light of day in Mountain Iron, Minnesota, named for its mountain of iron. Shortly after we married, Linda and I traveled there and walked to the edge of a mountain-size hole in the ground from where all the iron ore had gone. Empty foundations along the streets, their houses gone, testified that most of the people had gone too.

The old-as-the-Steinway generation make up most of the people I see—octogenarians, at the current limit of the human life span, babies in the Roaring Twenties. A birthday boy approaching his ninetieth birthday said, "It's good to be ninety. Most of the people I know die in their eighties." True. For the typical eighty-something in a nursing home, the average life span is two and a half years.

Had it not been for the family tie, Helen would have been my patient. She spent her final days in one of my nursing homes, sick and mopey. They called her depressed. I would have treated her if not for the family tie, and her family, Linda, didn't let my medical colleagues add an antidepressant to her long list of pills. Linda's grandmother also met her end in a nursing home back in the mythological era when families took care of their own. Linda thinks her family would have upheld traditional family values and taken her in, but her grandmother Hilda, a typical Finn, wanted to be left alone. First, she moved away from the farm, away from her bachelor son, Urho, into a small apartment in town. After her decline and entry into the nursing home, and well before the days of Wander-Guard, she would walk out the door and be found wandering aimlessly through the streets of Buhl, Minnesota.

For Hilda's daughter, Helen, a construction sleight of hand had transformed Linda's elementary school into a nursing home—going cradle to grave. It's a short walk—for those who can walk—from

Helen and her daughter's home to the nursing home. Linda walked that route to school with her kid brother every day.

Millions of stories like Helen's are happening to people every day. I hold some of their hands and bring what comfort I can to this generation, the parents of us boomers. I am in a unique position to hear their oral history of the twentieth century. An honor. But there's this: No matter how exciting or mundane the narrative arc of their lives, whether they were the CEO of a Fortune 500 company with one home in Greenwich and another in Bar Harbor or a life-long alcoholic loser dying with an already dead liver, they have all wound up in a corner of a hospital-style room with only a curtain for privacy. The CEO and the dead-liver man could be roomies. You're living in a public space where you can't lock your door and strangers walk by and see you lying helplessly in bed. You might be lying next to someone who spends his waking days screaming, "Help! Please help!" Or you might be the one screaming. You depend on the paid kindness of strangers. Some among us promote this thing called the culture of life. I write about the culture of life too—the department of disease, dying, and death.

Except for a month or two, Helen lived most of her life outside a nursing home. My mother died in the hospital, hours after collapsing in front of the TV munching an apple. Linda's father had only a few hospital hours before dying of his second stroke. Only my father had the full nursing home experience; an experience—given his dementia—of which he was mostly unaware. But even he spent most of his life on the outside. I have to remind myself that I'm seeing only a slice of life, even if it's the last slice.

My only direct contact with the people about whom I write is during their institutionalization. I have had no experience of their lives as they were slowly growing as old as our Steinway. My perspective is narrow and foreshortened—by what I see in the present and what they tell me about their past. My view is as distorted as any psychotherapist's.

I have worked with people of all ages but try to keep in mind that childhood is more than bed-wetting, night terrors, incest, school phobia, and self-mutilation. With adults, I learned that there's more than agoraphobia, compulsions, impotence, infidelity, and addiction. At the end of the life span, I see incontinence, delusions, depression, and unfocused rage. Had I known Helen only in a nursing home, and thought of her only as the person in the nursing home, I might have missed the teenage girl traveling alone with her girlfriend from a small mining town of mostly Finns to war work in Los Angeles, where she would encounter her Italian husband from New Haven, curiously replicating the journey her mother had made more than one hundred years ago with her girlfriend from her port town in northern Finland to the Mesabi Iron Range.

What I see before me is not all that there is.

That my father is not solely the angry man who tells me and all others to "get the hell out of here." That he was my father, who muddled through a varied life on more than one continent.

That Mrs. Henderson is not only the disheveled, shrunken lady with one somewhat good eye paired with a hollow socket who tells me her husband ran off with their new baby. That she studied at the Art Institute of Chicago.

That Mr. Lavelle is not only the paralyzed man who navigates his power wheelchair with puffs of air through a tube. That more than sixty years ago, he climbed the Pointe du Hoc cliff with his fellow Army Rangers on D-Day.

———

James Lavelle, sound of mind but not body, eighty-seven years old, sits most of his days in his air-powered wheelchair. He has had several strokes, but hung on tenaciously at home until his needs became too great for his third wife, only fifty-three. Mr. Lavelle shared the migratory ways of my mother-in-law. He grew up in Presque Isle, Maine, where his French-speaking parents had filtered down without papers from Quebec to work in the logging industry. Today, we complain about Mexicans streaming across our southern border, but undocumented entry is as American as apple pie. Samuel Goldwyn, for example, sailed to Nova Scotia in 1898, disembarked, walked hundreds of miles, and then crossed the U.S. border illegally before creating Hollywood—his American dream come to life on the silver screen. Some years later in 1939, James Lavelle, aged eighteen, left the logging life of his father behind and traveled with a friend to become a machinist in the ramped up war industry of the Connecticut River valley near the town of Vernon.

"I see you were at D-Day," I say. "You climbed the cliffs."

"Yeah, that was fun, but not as much as the boys had at Omaha Beach."

He's good at being an aw-shucks hero.

After the war, Lavelle went to the University of Connecticut on the GI Bill, became an engineer, and eventually bought the machine shop he worked at before his Army Ranger days. Illegal immigrant Goldwyn invented Hollywood; illegal immigrant Lavelle, a process for smoothing metal surfaces.

"Back in those days, UConn was still just a few brick buildings in the middle of farmland. Not like today, where it's high-rises stuck in the middle of housing developments."

His first wife, a student who became a teacher, was struck down by a drunk driver while she was picking up the mail from their roadside mailbox.

"Can you pour me a glass of water?"

He has limited use of his arms and hands, not enough to push a wheelchair, hence the propulsion by puffs of air. His three strokes have destroyed his body yet left him lucid and verbal. I pour the water, insert a straw, push aside the tube that motors the wheelchair, and put the drinking straw to his lips—a rare hands-on event for me.

His second wife, "a real beauty, but a cheat. She ran off on me, afraid I'd kill her, but I'm a kind of pacifist. I only kill people I don't know, Germans. Shows you how much she didn't know me. My real reaction: good riddance to bad garbage."

The History of the Peloponnesian War by Thucydides sits on his nightstand next to *A People's History of the United States* by Howard Zinn. After thirty years with the machine shop, Lavelle sold it and taught high school history in the ten years before his first stroke.

None of his wives had any children.

"I was hoping maybe with Joyce, my third one, even as old as I was, but the strokes killed that for me. She's a comfort in my old age. But I feel bad about it. I married her for her youth, but all I've given her is my old age."

At my next stop, I meet with Abigail Anscombe, another teacher, also in her eighties, also without children. She left her home in one of the tonier neighborhoods of Stamford, where her father was a banker, went to Smith College, and stayed on in Northampton, Massachusetts, never to return to Stamford until now. I lived in Northampton for six years, which I jokingly called the San Francisco of lesbianism. I wonder about Anscombe's sexuality, but that's none of my business. Next to her bed is a chess set. Too bad I can't hook her up with Sam Rosen. I could tell him I found him a game. But Anscombe resides too far away and is too far gone. She's terminally ill and has come home, which is where you go when there's no other place. I smile a hello to her and to her brother at her side before I shuffle down the hall to the room of Lenny McNair.

McNair is no ex-hero. He served in the war, but drove a truck far from the front lines. After the war, not skipping a beat, he continued to drive for the government, the postal service, for more than forty years. His wife is dead and his children have all moved away.

I'm waiting for him while someone wipes his bottom in the bathroom.

"Mr. McNair, do you have a family?"

"Yes, I do."

"Anyone comes to visit you?"

"No. I haven't talked to them in years."

"Where are they?"

"I think they're in Oklahoma."

"What's the date?"

"I don't pay attention to that type of thing."

"What's the name of this place?"

"Hellhole."

As I said, no matter the narrative arc of their lives, this is where much of the greatest generation is living. Their lives squeezed into five-digit diagnostic codes. I know it's wildly inaccurate, but sometimes I view the world as consisting of two kinds of people: those in nursing homes and those not yet in nursing homes. "That he not busy being born is busy dying," sang Bob Dylan.

It's easy for me to fixate on the Greatest Generation—most of the people I see—but they're transitory. If I were writing this ten years earlier, I'd be talking about the cohort born during World War I, children who survived the worldwide flu epidemic that killed fifty million, far more than the Great War's measly twenty. They were young adults at the height of the Depression, and some were exempt from World War II service because of family responsibilities. Both my parents were part of this generation. My father did serve in the war, but he was a decade older than most of his fellow draftees. Maybe that's why he became a sergeant. They even wanted him to go to officer candidate school. But he declined, knowing that "second louies," as he called them, had the highest casualty rate. Good thing for me.

Ten years from now, if I'm still in this line of work, it will be Depression babies—sometimes called the Silent Generation. These were the kids who tended victory gardens and collected scrap metal to support the war effort. Later, they would get the dubious honor of fighting the Korean War.

And twenty years from now it will be my boomer generation. Will the Beatles songbook replace the Glenn Miller sing-along? Will I nod off in my wheelchair in the face of an endless YouTube loop? Will fading memories be prodded by trivia games about *Rootie Kazootie* and *The Brady Bunch*? Will a group of us be wondering why we can't get a hit of weed, rather than the glass of wine some of my patients agitate for today?

Traveling between nursing homes the other day, I stopped for gas and spied someone not yet in a nursing home, reminding me of my distorted view of old age. There at the next pump was a gent—maybe late seventies, early eighties—gassing up his Lexus

LS. I looked it up. They start at $61,500. Eyeing his cream-color leisure suit—they still make those?—and white shoes, I was polite enough not to remind him it was after Labor Day. And I asked myself, "Who am I calling old?" The leisure-suited Lexus man and millions of others are out there quite independently living their lives of quiet desperation.

I shouldn't forget the octogenarian triathletes, eighty-nine-year-old Walter Cronkite sailing his boat, Pete Seeger still singing, Harry Bernstein publishing his well-reviewed debut novel at age ninety-seven, and sixty-eight-year-old Melvin Cate, bank robber. Nor should I forget my Aunt Estelle, born at the beginning of the last century in the Ukraine, mugged in front of her Brooklyn home and injured because she fought the muggers off.

There's a game I like to play that I can play anywhere. Let's play it at the local convenience store. In my upscale neighborhood, I've been told, it is the only sign of life at three a.m., when the other local burghers and I are tucked safely in bed. This gas station convenience store is the crossroads for all types of humans, including stickup artists who favor it for its close proximity to the interstate for a getaway. That happens when the cops aren't grabbing a coffee and flirting with the clerks. And there are the Yalies piling snacks on the counter for their youthful bodies. In the line in front of me, not at three a.m., is a fortysomething woman, much fatter than I, and at least a foot shorter. She asks for a couple of packs of Marlboros. On the counter she has placed a Milky Way, a family-size bag of chips, a nondiet Pepsi, a half-gallon of whole milk, and a loaf of white bread—Wonder Bread (invented in 1921, two years before

Helen and the Steinway were born). She almost forgets, while pocketing her uncounted change, to ask for ten dollars' worth of lottery tickets.

Doctors, I've heard, play a variation of this game. They might look at me hanging onto a strap on a bus, see the way I'm standing, and guess that I have lower-back pain. I'm looking at the woman in front of me and guessing she'll be lucky to make it to seventy without being in a nursing home, probably with type 2, non-insulin-dependent diabetes, hypertension, high cholesterol, and chronic obstructive pulmonary disease.

As I leave the store, watching her drive off in her battered Chevette, I notice a runner go by. He's making good time. As a former marathoner myself, I estimate he's on a six-minute-per-mile pace. He's imperially slim, and I estimate that barring any disease unrelated to fitness—Parkinson's or Alzheimer's—he's good for a lifetime outside the nursing home.

Me? My marathoning days are long gone, but I still exercise. Although I could lose more than a few pounds, on the plus side I quit smoking more than twenty-five years ago, with only a one-year lapse along the way. On the negative side, quitting is not as good as never having smoked. I had a rare tumor and the doctors didn't get all of it, and told me it could kill me someday. But just as likely not. My genes are decent. My mother made it into her eighties, and my father almost hit ninety, albeit with dementia. I have a reasonable shot at not being in the nursing home until I'm older than the Steinway is today. I also have a reasonable shot at keeling over before I'm frail or demented enough for the home. None of this means that my right knee won't ache when I stand up and it bears my weight.

Being in the nursing home at the age of the Steinway is par for the course. But to be there in your seventies is a bitter failure.

I'm at St. Albans Green. It's not bucolic. It's inner city, red brick, early twentieth century. If it weren't a nursing home, it could have been my Brooklyn elementary school, P.S. 169, except it's not six stories tall and there's no playground. Shiftless locals loiter on the corner exchanging envelopes with hands reaching out of cars. I'm meeting with Mrs. Piscitelle. She's seventy-three, gravely ill, sad, and worried about when she's going home. She and her husband were lifelong factory workers working for a subcontractor that built obscure parts for the Connecticut defense industry. They live in a working-class neighborhood in an aging port town of neat little houses, picket fences, and impatiens that stemmed the tide of welfare houses at one end but is losing the battle against gentrification at the other. I enter the room and there's an energetic, thin but not frail gent sitting on the one chair. He's not wearing the anachronistic leisure suit of the Lexus driver but jeans and a work shirt.

"Hi, I'm Ira Rosofsky, a psychologist. Are you Mrs. Piscitelle's husband? They wanted me to see her."

"They're weighing her."

As he's speaking, an aide wheels in Agnes Piscitelle. Her husband's thin, she's pathologically frail. Pancreatic cancer. She's only seventy-three.

"Could I meet with your wife for a bit?"

"Want me to leave?"

"Just for a little while. I'll be happy to talk with you after."

It's an article of professional faith that it's often better to begin without the family around. The physical presence of a spouse could influence what's said.

"In your own words, why are you here?"

"It's my darn foot. It's fractured, and I need to get on my feet before I go home."

She does have a foot problem, but it's not a fracture, and it's not the problem.

"My husband's mad at me. He wants us to keep doing stuff like going to the casinos and bus tours to Canada. That was the plan. He might have to do it by himself. But I don't think he wants to."

It's not clear to me if she knows how gravely ill she is. She puts all the weight of it on her foot. That might get better. The foot is her excuse for not being able to lead the life they had planned. There are no children, so they've had to take consolation only from each other, with a dash of extended family thrown in. I have a sad image of Mr. Piscitelle, not on the foliage bus through New England to meet the Bar Harbor ferry to Halifax but alone on the Fung Wah bus to Mohegan Sun, alone at the slots, with no one to share his booty at the buffet. Mrs. Piscitelle might make it home for a bit, to be in the care of her as yet able husband, worrying about his resentment: "My husband's mad at me." Or she might not even make it home, lingering in confinement while Mr. Piscitelle spends his mornings at a diner reading the *New Haven Register*, drinking coffee, and stepping outside for a smoke as he scratches at his lottery tickets. I find him in front of the building. He offers me a Marlboro. I offer him the opportunity to chat. He replies, "Thanks for stopping, Doc." With a perfunctory "She's unhappy. She wants to get home," he shrugs and walks back in.

When you're seventy-three in the nursing home, you are there before your time. You're the fat lady buying cigarettes, whole milk, and Wonder Bread in front of me at the convenience store. Or you got dealt a bad hand, not at the casino but at life. Mrs. Piscitelle is not the smoker in the family, and pancreatic cancer has nothing to do with that, anyway. You might be Senator Pete Domenici, planning to run yet again but giving it up for degenerative frontal-lobe brain disease, which causes a type of dementia. If Domenici weren't one of those senatorial multimillionaires rich enough for 24/7 nursing care at home, he would wind up in a nursing home too.

No matter how old you are, it's too soon to lose your independence. If you're seventy-three with slim prospects of returning home—the pill is more bitter.

"Are you basically satisfied with your life?" I ask off the Beck Geriatric Depression Scale.

"I was until I came here," a typical answer.

Sometimes a seventy-year-old will add, "I'm surrounded by all these old people."

I agree. I'm over sixty, but still of the mind-set where I see youth in me and old age in others—often where I have no right to. I regularly refer to people my age or younger as old. They look old to me. I look in the mirror, still see me, and nothing that's old like them. Familiarity breeds familiarity. When I looked at my old parents, I saw, as always, my mother and father. With my self-imagined forever-young persona, I chat up young Yalies. In my mind, I'm flirting. In their minds, I'm Gramps.

Among the younger residents in nursing homes—who, nevertheless, by my mind's trickery always look old to me—is a mixed bag of people.

Ms. Jennifer Petrowski sits in her room at an assisted-living center. It's a nice room. Never married, she relies on the kindness of nieces, nephews, sisters, brothers, cousins. Their photos line the dresser. The TV is loud and blaring, but she stares at it blankly.

She remembers the big picture: that she cleaned houses and eventually had a little business. She hired other people to help her clean, bought an annuity that pays for the assisted living. Lucky her.

The little picture is a bit hazy.

"What town is this?" I ask.

"Connecticut."

"What's the name of this place?"

"I don't know. My home."

"Who's the president?"

"Carter."

"How old are you?"

Here I get coyness, or seem to.

"Forty-seven."

But she is sixty-three, with early-onset Alzheimer's, plus there's the breast cancer and the obesity.

I look at her and it's hard to imagine that she is my age, my generation. She doesn't seem the type, but she could have been at Woodstock with me. I might have danced beside her at a disco. She might have voted for Reagan, while I was voting for all my loser Democrats. But now she has a much steeper hill on which to decline than the long, slow glide path I imagine for myself.

The younger you are in the nursing home, the more dire your straits—another Rosofsky law.

Tucked away in rural hill country is Ludford Bridge Manor. You could easily miss the small, discreet sign off the back-road, two-lane blacktop. Charles Stegley is forty-three. He has amyotrophic lateral sclerosis (ALS), Lou Gehrig's disease, but I doubt he'd say he's the luckiest man alive. The odds of winning the Powerball lottery are one in eighty million. In the United States, your odds of getting ALS are much better, only one in sixty thousand. There are five thousand newly diagnosed cases each year and thirty thousand people with the condition at any given time—a small number, which brings no comfort to Stegley.

Nursing homes are not only for the aged. If you win a negative lottery and get ALS, Parkinson's, or multiple sclerosis, or get hit by a car or fall out of a window, you could be young in a nursing home.

Stegley, married without children, had a nice little business, a fact reflected in the many books lining the walls of his room. A college dropout, he loved to read and buy books, mostly used, mostly from tag sales and dusty back bins at used-book stores. He thought he was just being thrifty, but a friend told him his first edition of *To Kill a Mockingbird* might be worth something. He found out it was worth over a thousand dollars. That got his attention.

"Ira, if you ever want to quit the shrink business," he told me, "you could do worse than hanging out at tag sales and buying whatever first edition you see."

Stegley became an early adopter of eBay, selling his books for fun and profit—which was a comfortable enough life—but suddenly he started tripping and falling. He slurred his speech. He was diagnosed with ALS at age thirty-nine. For a couple of years he hung on at home, but eventually, he was unable to walk, get dressed, and or feed himself—Activities of Daily Living. His wife, a successful realtor, decided he needed more than her, and he got less of her. He's been at Ludford Bridge for two years.

He's in one of those wheelchairs that look like recliners on wheels. It eases the pain in his back, which is not strong enough to support him in an upright position. He's fed and diapered by others, but ALS, which varies greatly, has left his speech reasonably intact—slurred only enough to make him sound like a cartoon character.

"She's only thirty-five. I didn't get married for a long time, and when I did I made sure to marry someone young enough for kids."

This reminds me of my own situation, married at forty-two to someone ten years younger. I get to be with someone always younger than whatever old age I'm at, and she gets to feel younger. It's a good deal for both of us, except for the probable years of widowhood that lie before her—unless she comes to think that's a good deal. Neither of us talks much about the future. Even if I make it to ninety, for her, there will likely be years without me.

"I'm surprised she hasn't left me yet," Stegley says without bitterness. "Maybe she hasn't met the one yet."

"Maybe she loves you," I suggest.

There are shelves around the room bearing the weight of Stegley's remaining inventory. I see an eclectic mélange. There's *In Cold Blood*. "He was a childhood friend of Lee's, so after her one and only book got me started I had to have one of his." Nearby is *Valley of the Dolls*. "For reading, it's trash. For selling, I could get five hundred, more than it's worth. Jacqueline signed it." In his mind, he is on a first-name basis with the authors. Some of his gems are in a locked cabinet. *Leaves of Grass*. "It's only a second edition, but what can you do?" Next to Whitman are the first paperback editions of *The Great Gatsby* and *On the Road*. "The fiftieth anniversary of Kerouac is coming up. It will be worth more."

Stegley may not be able to wait for that. His savings are running out. And although there's a computer in the corner, he can't easily use it; only when his wife has the time can he work on selling off his inventory.

"I think she's a little ticked I didn't transfer my assets to her long enough ago so they won't be eaten by Medicaid. But she's making enough from selling the houses, so she doesn't need it. She doesn't have bookselling in her blood. My business dies with me."

So Stegley is spending down at a young age. His six-figure savings will go for the nursing home, so will the proceeds from his current sales. Under the regulations, he was allowed to buy himself the fancy custom wheelchair, the computer in his room, some nice clothes, and the big-screen TV. When spending down, Medicaid allows you to buy personal-use items, which are not counted as part of your total allowable assets of about $2,000. When my father was spending down, we outfitted him with a complete new wardrobe and new furniture for his already subsidized apartment. But Stegley's books will have to go. They're business inventory, not personal effects. The Medicaid regs say it's perfectly okay for Stegley to read *On the Road*, but it can't be the first paperback edition. Their not unreasonable attitude is, "We're paying Stegley's $75,000 annual bill, and he gets to keep $2,000 in the bank."

Leaving aside the fact that it would be cheaper for Medicaid to find him a personal assistant so he could continue his business and pay for his own nursing home care, the authorities at Ludford Bridge will be happy to see the books go. They make noises about unsafe clutter, but that's likely beside the point. These are institutions, after all, that rely on routine and regimentation. They're at a loss about what to do with personalized lives. Once he sells off his inventory and is on Medicaid, Stegley will lose his private room and move to a nondescript one with a stranger.

Stegley is one of the sprinkling of young people I see who, for a variety of reasons, can't be at home. I wonder about Stegley's wife. What's in it for her? Is it love? Is there someone on the side comforting her through the ordeal ahead? Idle thoughts for me. It's really none of my business.

I've met her. Attractive, blond, but thickening at the waist. She's solicitous, but takes no nonsense. Tends to tell him he's trying too hard. He should take it easy. Maybe she likes her life the way it is. Not every woman wants a spouse and children. With Charles, she sees what "for better or worse" can actually mean.

He tells me she loves her career and hands me her card. She says it's a shame they can't afford 24/7 care for him at home. He confides, "She hates it when I pee my pants. Joan's definitely not a diaper person."

I wonder how Linda or I would handle it if, God forbid, something happened to one of us. And I realize as I stare candidly into the mirror that it's no longer a question of a bad thing happening to a young person. I joke about old farts, but I'm one too. An *alter kaker* as my ancestors would say—an "old shit."

Not every young person in a nursing home has an early-onset degenerative disease—Parkinson's, multiple sclerosis, Lou Gehrig's. I see my share of those, but there's a whole other class of young ones, almost hidden.

When I lived in Northampton, there stood Tan Man on the corner of Main and Pleasant, so-called because he wore shorts and no shirt in any kind of weather. Nearby stood Winter Coat Man in a heavy blue parka in any kind of weather.

Their emergence on the street came at the end of a century-plus incarceration of the chronically mentally ill, the rebellious, and the eccentric in state hospitals across our land. The reformist fervor of the abolitionist movement also infused the founding of hospitals as a response to the treatment of the insane, whom Dorothea Dix found "in cages, stalls, pens! Chained, naked, beaten with rods, and lashed into obedience."

Three years before the Civil War, in 1858, Massachusetts established the Northampton Lunatic Hospital based on "moral treatment"—a regimen of fresh air, dignified labor, and cultural pursuits. At its high-water mark in 1950, there were twenty-five hundred patients in a self-sufficient city-state that spanned 538 acres—almost a square mile—with slaughterhouses, agriculture, and housing for the staff as well as the patients. The staff grew old surrounded by their families; the cloistered patients grew old irrevocably separated from their families.

This high-water mark was the beginning of the end. Moral treatment—along with Freudianism and shock treatment—met their match in the marriage of the chemical restraint revolution and the civil rights movement. Reformers wanted to mainstream the insane, and it seemed possible—as long as they took their meds.

Gradually, they emptied out the state hospital. In 1976, the Commonwealth of Massachusetts signed a judicial consent decree, agreeing to deinstitutionalize the remaining five hundred patients and shut the place down. Thus Tan Man and Winter Coat Man—the perpetually warm and the perpetually cold—came to stand together on the corner of Pleasant and Main.

But not all the tan men are standing on the corner watching the supposedly sane go by.

I'm sitting in the dining room of Northallerton Hall. It's next to the hospital in a midsize town. It's utilitarian. Formica tables. None of the white linen I find in the high-end assisted-living facilities. I'm at one table writing notes, a group of residents at the next table. Four women, all young enough to be my children.

"Now what's the Zyprexa? For the depression?" asks a cadaverously slim one.

"No, that's the Lexapro," replies a morbidly obese one in a wheelchair. "The Zyprexa is to help you think more clearly."

"I thought the Zyprexa was supposed to help me with my voices."

"That too, and if you don't hear voices you might be able to think more clearly."

They go on, discussing and debating their various drugs—the minutiae of various tranquilizers, the effects of the various antipsychotics on auditory versus visual hallucinations. I continue writing my notes, with one ear tuned in. Maybe I could learn something. These people have had more experience with psychopharmacology than me. Even if they don't know what they're talking about, they sound like they do.

Here's what happened to the deinstitutionalized.

It was easy to empty out the institutions. Just open the doors. It was harder to build community-based institutions. Plus it was expensive. For a while, you could ignore the street crazies. It was cheaper than funding group homes with an expensive professional staff. For many former inmates of state hospitals, their pharmacist became their community mental health program. But then a lightbulb rather than a voice went on in someone's head. These crazies have Medicaid. Why don't we put them in nursing homes?

Joyce Gandolph has the half of the room by the window. By the door is an octogenarian with not much of a life. The old lady's side of the room is bare and unadorned. Never married. No visitors. No photos. Joyce's side of the room is charitably describable as overflowing. It looks as if a bag lady who used to push a shopping cart down the street piled high with overloaded garbage bags suddenly found her clean, well-lighted place. Joyce styles herself a poet and there are heaps of notebooks along with the other detritus from her life—stuffed animals without stuffing, jewelry boxes without jewelry, a bone-china demitasse cup—covering every surface in the room, including the floor. I wonder how the demitasse cup—I almost tripped over it—survived life on the streets. I turn it over and there's a Limoges mark.

Joyce, in her early fifties, says that as long as she takes her meds she doesn't hear voices. She hasn't talked to her daughter in years and doesn't know her whereabouts. To hear Joyce tell the story, her daughter called her collect from Texas three years ago. She didn't accept the charges and hasn't heard from her since. Joyce is a former Bostonian. Her brother, she tells me—and I have no reason to disbelieve her—is a semiprominent art restorer. "He specializes in pottery," and I speculate that could be the provenance of the Limoges. Her father owned a luggage shop downtown. She attended one of the many colleges in Boston but dropped out to marry her husband, an attorney, just before moving to Connecticut. Shortly after, she gave birth to her daughter, and a couple of years later her husband died in a car crash. "He drank quite a bit, and I was already hearing voices. One told me to kill my kid, but my parents took her away. They're dead now. Served them right." It is doubtful her artisan brother could afford anything more than Northallerton for Joyce, if he cared. Joyce says he calls her occasionally and visits "once in a blue moon."

Northallerton is full of people drifting away from their families, living in reduced circumstances, sliding down the social hierarchy. They—and in many cases their abandoned or neglected children—are lost to the middle class. The downward drift of Joyce Gandolph is the downside of the American dream. In these reduced circumstances, many aspire to little more than an exit pass from Northallerton. Others see Northallerton as a reasonable end point.

From one resident I hear, "It's winter now, too cold, but when it gets warm, I hope I find an apartment." Another attests, "This is better than living in my car."

At Northallerton, which has mostly psychiatric patients (many other nursing homes have a sprinkling), I see what happened to the state hospital and the dream of deinstitutionalization. The chronically mentally ill were not integrated into the community. Neither did we leave them in peace to be bare-chested on the corner of Pleasant and Main, or squeegeeing your windshield at the entrance to the Holland Tunnel. Community integration (like school integration) remains a dream. The state hospital is still with us, but in the privatized form of Northallerton.

Visit the grounds of Northampton State today, and you will see mostly derelict, crumbling red brick buildings—Shakespeare's "bare, ruined choirs." Thirty years after the consent decree closing the joint, signs of life other than weeds are emerging. Some clever realtor, maybe Mrs. Stegley, has rechristened the place as Hospital Hill. The latest master plan, after years of dead ends, calls for a mix of affordable housing, market-priced housing, offices, light industrial use, and assisted living. And 15 percent of the housing will be for the mentally ill. Maybe not Tan Man, I heard he died, but others like him will come full circle into the Hospital Hill set-aside housing.

I'm not sure if Tan Man's end was happy, but there are some happily-ever-after stories in nursing homes.

There is a kind of natural selection, a survival of the fittest, in life and in nursing homes. When I was an ingénue in this line of work and they referred someone to me who was over ninety, I instinctively recoiled, thinking it would be a chore to talk to one so old—that they would be deafer, blinder, and more confused. To my surprise and delight, the opposite is true. Very old folks, people in their nineties, can be haler and heartier than their mostly younger fellow residents. Some of the very old have outlived their caretakers. Others, improbably, are on a round-trip ticket home.

Consider Sean Hanrahan. When I met him, he was shortly to become one of the few humans alive to have had the personal enjoyment of the last two Red Sox baseball championships—1918 and 2004.

On my way to his room at rural Meldon Meadows, the nurse pulled me aside and warned me he was cranky, unfriendly, and in a world of pain. A fit ninety-six, he fell off a ladder while hanging a picture and broke his leg. At that age, a fracture is usually a one-way ticket to institutional confinement. But Sean was determined to get home.

Born in Boston, 1908, he wasn't at the 1918 World Series clincher. He was poor, plus there were only 42,000 seats.

"I didn't even hear it on the radio. There was no radio. I heard the newsboys down the street hawking the late-edition extra."

I met Sean on my fifty-eighth birthday, October 27, 2004—almost old enough to cash in my IRA but still too young for Medicare. Sean and all the other residents provide me with—apologies to Wordsworth—intimations of my own mortality.

I also remember that date because in the evening the Sox were to finish their four-game sweep of the Cardinals. Despite the nurse's warning, Sean was in a celebratory, talkative mood—wearing his Bosox hat.

"I'm a bit unhappy I can't be at the game. My grandson told me if they ever made it this far, he'd take me. But I got my TV right here, and the nurse has a beer cooling for me in their fridge."

That night, stuffed with New Haven pizza, I'm sitting in front of my TV—birthday cake on my lap, more than a shot of Balvenie DoubleWood single malt in a goblet by my side. Long-suffering Mets fan that I am, at least it's not the Yankees, I think, as I watch the Red Sox get off their eighty-six-year-old schneid, completing their four-game sweep of the Cardinals—their first since their last championship over the forever hapless Cubs back in 1918.

The following week, I'm back, and Sean is gone. My heart skips a beat, but he's not dead. He's home. Even at ninety-six, life can go on.

If I live long enough—I would be ninety-six in 2042—I too will have a baseball story of the previous century for some eager whipper-snapper. It will sound equally quaint to the ears of someone who will be long past computers, iPhones, and HDTV.

I was only eight (not ten like Hanrahan) when the Brooklyn Dodgers won their only World Series. We took our baseball seriously in Brooklyn. No need to play hooky to follow the series. They wheeled those newfangled TVs right into the classrooms. I'm not sure whether watching baseball fulfilled the TVs' purported educational role. Although I did have a TV by 1955, I belonged to the very last generation not to automatically have one as a birthright. We didn't get our Andrea TV in its beautiful mahogany cabinet until I was six. If the game wasn't over when the school bell rang, no problem: walking home we could follow the game from the radios and TVs through the open windows. The Bums—as we affectionately called them—clinched the series with a 2–0 complete game by Johnny Podres. Outside my house, a Yankee was hanged in effigy (good and evil clearly defined) from the street lamp, and who could sleep with all the firecrackers, cherry bombs, and ash cans—even guns—going off through the night?

Pete Hamill would write, "In Brooklyn that day, it was the Liberation of Paris, Vee Jay Day, New Year's Day all rolled into one."

I would go on to learn at the still young age of eleven that good and evil are not so easily defined when the Dodgers went west along with my naïveté in 1958, never to return, except as the enemy of my newfound love, the Mets. Even though I was able to give my heart, on the rebound, to another, my eyes were opened wide after the Dodgers helped plant the seeds of the cynical detachment with which I continue to live today.

I don't know if Sean lives today, but it's not a stretch to believe he lived to see the Sox win yet another championship in 2007 somewhere not in a nursing home and living without cynicism forever in the moment. His Sox never left him.

5 BED, BATHS, AND BEYOND BINGO

Daily Life at the End of Life

Were I Christo—gift-wrapper of buildings, arrayer of uncount-able umbrellas and gates—I'd do wheelchair art. Nurs-ing home staffs are inadvertently Christoesque. They array found objects—wheelchairs with people in them—in lines snaking down the hall waiting for the dining room, in circles to pass a ball around for recreation, as a chorus at the nursing station, fitted like Tetris pieces into elevators. The residents themselves serve up a kind of random Brownian array, folk-art Pollocks one and all, moving in unpredict-able directions. I could tie paintbrushes to their wheelchairs—their wanderings trailing works of art along the floors. I could pull out my cell phone—in facilities that allow cell phones—and, violator of all things HIPAA, take snapshots and submit them to *American Photo*. Call it something fancy like Dementia Stochastica.

I'm sitting in a lounge, writing notes. A resident rolls in and rear-ranges the shelf of unread *Reader's Digest Condensed Books* before reaching for my papers. Some neurons are firing off telling her it's a mess, clean it up.

"Hi. How ya doin'? No, that's mine."

She rolls off, no paintbrush trailing behind her.

Back in the 1980s, a group of researchers sat around observing nursing home residents in their natural setting. They had elaborate charts and forms in which they were planning to mark down each type of activity for each resident at various times through the day. It must have been boring. Most residents spent most of their time in the felicitously named category of "null behavior." In response to studies such as these, the federal government—arbiter of all things nursing home—mandated in an infelicitously named law, The Omnibus Budget Reconciliation Act of 1987 (OBRA), that nursing homes "support residents in preferred activity." OBRA, in many ways, established the landscape of the nursing home I see today. OBRA brought us individual care plans, mandated physical and occupational therapy, formalized minimum data sets and activities of daily living—the MDSs and the ADLs—required state inspectors to speak to residents and families as well as staff, and resident councils—the student governments of nursing homes. In addition to providing employment for thousands of new worker bees who spend no time with residents—such as the MDS tabulators and care-planning coordinators, OBRA made provisions for quality of life in addition to quantity of care. It decreed that there would be an activity director specifically charged with filling the recreational time of the residents. Fast-forward twenty years, and, sadly, for all the activity about activity, recent studies also find the residents engaging in "no observable behavior."

To be fair, are those of us on the outside—both old and young—much more active?

Karl Marx promised that the Communist man would "hunt in the morning, fish in the afternoon, rear cattle in the evening, and criticize after dinner." Well, that never happened, but even in the rapacious robber-baron era of the nineteenth century—the Gilded Age—we were all quite active. The late Jean Mayer, nutritionist and president of Tufts University, described the life of a typical nineteenth-century sedentary office worker. He would wake up at dawn, chop wood, and fetch water from the well before walking several miles to his office, where he would stand working at his desk for ten to twelve hours. Then he would walk home and chop more wood, along with other physically demanding labors. And this was the sedentary man.

Today, for the twenty-first-century man, sedentary is sedentary: null behavior for us all.

Each year, the Bureau of Labor Statistics publishes the American Time Use Survey, which summarizes average daily activities for both men and women. Among the findings from the 2006 survey: employed men worked an average of 8.4 hours, women, 7.7. At home, men and women averaged one hour per day in household activities such as cooking, cleaning, and paying bills. Sleep killed 7.6 hours, leaving the remainder for leisure or child care. Although women interacted with their children for 1.2 hours—activities ranging from bathing them to storybook time—men managed only a stingy twenty minutes. I wonder what this says to those who advocate father-present families as essential for healthy child development. The present father is largely absent. I wonder how much moral and cognitive tutelage our kids get from watching their fathers spend three hours each day surfing the Internet or watching TV. I guess they learn to surf the Internet and watch TV.

That's the working man and woman. What about older, retired Americans? Are they finally getting around to *Remembrance of Things Past*?

The average person aged sixty-five to seventy-four—the Golden Years—has about seven daily hours of leisure time. More than half of that goes into watching TV. There's less than an hour for reading—likely the newspaper—half an hour for the computer or games, twenty minutes for some kind of exercise, less than an hour for socializing, and almost an hour for "relaxing and thinking"— sounds like a nap to me. And these are the averages. Many older Americans have a meal and then spend most of their leisure time in front of the TV—in other words, engaging in no measurable activity. Same as in the nursing home.

Sobering and instructive numbers. Could I be all wrong about nursing home banality? Could it just be an extension of the normal routine of the older (and younger) American—but locked away with room service?

If I look at it in this way, I could maybe find contentment with life in a nursing home. If I couldn't swing a private room, I'd try for a bed by the window. Staff wouldn't always be walking by my bed to tend to the guy by the window. I'd be the guy by the window. I'd want a roommate with moderate dementia—pleasantly confused. I'd want him to be what we call redirectable. I'd tell him to wander off, giving me some privacy. Too much profound dementia and he'd be high maintenance—plenty of staff in the room diapering, feeding, medicating, restraining. Mild dementia, and he'd want to talk nonsense all the time. I'd know how to work the system. Nobody would bother me, because I'd be a nice and compliant unsqueaky wheel. Lots of yes sirs, and yes ma'ams. I'd mouth the heavy tranquilizers and spit them in the toilet. "Such a sweet old man," I'd hear them murmur. And they would leave sweet old me alone. I for one would catch up on my reading. I might actually crack open *Remembrance of Things Past*. I'd read all of Jane Austen again, but for fun not for credit. For something light, I'd work in Sue Grafton from A to whatever. Maybe she'll have Z done by then—or even have gone on to *AA Is for Alcohol-*

ics Anonymous. On nice days, I'd sit in the sun affecting a wide straw hat—maybe take up smoking again. I'd chat up the nurses. But no pinching. It almost sounds like one of the plausibly Mittyesque lives I imagine when the kids and the wife are too much. Maybe I'd write a bit, but for art and posterity, not for commercial success. Every day, I'd take a nap or two, and there would be no leftover tasks when I woke up just in time for dinner. No garbage to take out. No dogs to walk. No one to yell at. No one to yell at me. I'd be Burgess Meredith in *The Twilight Zone*—the sole survivor of a nuclear holocaust, who wanted only to read without the bother of a wife or boss, who finds his paradise in a library just before he steps on his glasses. But I'd take good care of my glasses. I'd have the nurse keep a spare for me. "Such a sweet old man." My eyes would follow her butt as she exited.

It is possible to look at the institution slantwise and game the system so it becomes a sanctuary where you do what you want and nobody bothers you. Unfortunately, if you are sound enough to enjoy it, they might not let you in. Yossarian stumbling over Catch-23. You might have to break a hip, be unable to breathe or think, and where's the enjoyment in that?

And there's this. It's easy for harsh retributive Puritans to condemn soft prisons—Club Fed with TVs, weight rooms, swimming pools, putting greens. But if you get lost in an idyll of the nursing home, ask yourself if you would prefer to be locked up in the Plaza with room service, free honor bar, crystal glass, Spode china, and percale sheets never able to leave for a walk in Central Park so beautiful through your window. Or would you prefer your unlocked hovel, able to walk outside into your slummy neighborhood whenever you had the inclination?

If the gilded cage has no appeal, you don't want to be in a nursing home.

I'm not sure how my mother would have come down on this one. She got a taste of the gilded cage. A few years before she died, when she was eighty-one, her doctors replaced a leaky heart valve. She planned everything in advance. The date for the surgery. The hundred phone calls to my brother and me making sure we would be at the hospital. And the post-op rehab—no slip and fall and a last-minute pressured move to an available bed.

Burke Rehabilitation Hospital, founded 1915 in White Plains, New York, is "12 neoclassical buildings and a series of graceful colonnades—all with a view of the surrounding countryside." Thomas Jefferson, fresh from Monticello, could have designed the joint. It's not an institution, not a facility. It's a campus. No long-term dementia here. If you have heart surgery, a stroke, brain damage, an amputation, knee or hip replacement—and you can reserve a room in advance—this might be the place for you. Well before they opened her heart, my mother knew she would be at Burke.

When I visited her there, she seemed quite serene. Maybe it was her weakened state taking her edge off, but she wore a smile my whole visit. Walking down the hall, residents and staff all saying hello. They wait on you hand and foot—literally and metaphorically. There was a fine meal, and she waved greetings to the other ladies and gents with whom she usually had dinner. She never looked better. I sensed she missed it all when, after discharge, I'd call and again hear, "I'm glad somebody finally called. I didn't know if my voice was still working."

For me, after they cut out most of my tumor and removed my collarbone ("You don't really need it"—easy for my doc to say), I get none of the luxury treatment. My surgeon tells me to go swimming. After weeks of splashing around and still the pain, he refers me to outpatient rehab. It's Gaylord—a Burke competitor. Perfectly first rank, but I don't go to the luxe inpatient facility. I have my sessions at a satellite location that looks like a warehouse. A physiatrist—the doctor specialist who is the lord of all rehab—examines me and laughs at the idea of swimming as rehab for a frozen shoulder.

"That's the worst thing he could advise you to do. But he's only a surgeon."

As an innocent bystander—but the one with the tumor—as a patient visiting many specialists, I got a lot of that. The docs using me as a sounding board to mock their colleagues. "What does he know about rehab? He's only a surgeon." I dutifully obey the physiatrist lady, and it's no more young things in tight Speedos for me to ogle at during community swim at the high school pool. Instead, I get Ken the physical therapist manipulating my shoulder's range of motion. I get to pedal a kind of bicycle contraption, but using my arms. Then I go into the gym and pump iron under close supervision. The only eye candy is wounded women in leotards on stair-climbers.

It's not always accurate, but it's sometimes useful to think of old age as a rewind of childhood. You go from walking to walking with a walker to sitting in a chair with wheels to lying in a bed not able to sit up at all. You go from feeding yourself to having someone feed you solid food and then liquids (but no breast milk) to intravenous—an analogue of the umbilical cord.

In some nursing homes, there are day-care centers. True cradle to grave, a terrific idea. Bring your child to work and view her through the picture windows lying on a cot napping away before you walk down the hall and see eighty-year-olds napping away too. Some of the residents, not napping, wheel over and watch the kids. Are they reflecting on the arc of life—as I am? When the babies and toddlers wake and play, it's spontaneous. No OBRA. No mandates.

Someone cleverly called play the work of childhood. This is a recent idea, a twentieth-century idea. Previously, for most children, work was the work of childhood. Quite early in life, you had to put aside childish things and become a man.

In 1932, the psychologist Mildred Parten outlined four stages of child's play. First, there is unoccupied play, when the child is, in effect, engaged in no observable behavior. The child may be aimlessly looking around, moving in no particular direction. Next, the child engages in solitary play, happily playing independently, trying to fit square pegs in round holes. He or she is playing but unconcerned about anyone else. This is followed by parallel play. Children still play by themselves, but side by side. There's minimal interaction. A child might try to grab another child's toy, but that's about it. There is a kind of group-think in this parallel play. One minute children might all be building block towers, the next playing with puppets—alone but together. The last stage of child play is cooperative play. Rather than solitary builders of block towers side by side, they form construction crews.

Reverse this and you can sketch out dementia's decline. Playing together. Playing side by side. Playing alone. Babbling and drooling on your own.

Despite this seemingly natural progression—or retrogression— despite a population that has had a lifetime of living on its own, OBRA mandated, rather vaguely, that "nursing homes support residents' engagement in preferred activities." Enter the activity director. For people of a certain age, such as myself, the term "activity director" brings to mind *The Love Boat* (always pronounced "the loooooove boat") and perky Julie McCoy. The recycling of faded stars through guest bits on that TV show inspires me to a sequel, foibles and high jinks in the nursing home—call it *Ship of Fools* or *Voyage of the Damned*—bringing back some truly ancient mariners with me as the star—the hapless staff psychologist, Doc, with the activity director played by the now fifty-three-year-old Lauren Tewes.

She would more or less fit the activity director demographic. As with most jobs in the home, it's predominantly female. But most of the activity directors are white, whereas most of the CNAs are black or Latino. Does this mean anything? Does it mean that people of color are okay to clean your body, but not to facilitate recreational fun? It's probably not racism but networking. Word somehow gets back to a community that this is the opportunity for you. It's the reason why Linda's relatives came to Mountain Iron, Minnesota, from Oulu, Finland, and my relatives wound up on the Lower East Side of Manhattan from Latichev, Ukraine. Word gets out to a community that there's a job that has benefits, a salary greater than Wal-Mart, and a modicum of a professional status. There are your CNAs. Word gets out to another community that you can play bingo with old people and not have to clean up their messes, and there are your activity directors.

But maybe there's a bit more. Becoming a CNA does not generally require a college degree, not even a two-year associate's degree. Generally, you get on-the-job training with some coursework thrown in to earn certification. Only seventy-five hours of training is the minimum standard.

Activity directors require at least a bit of college. OBRA 1987 mandates that activity departments be headed up by an "activity professional." Although there are certificate programs that do not require even an associate's degree, you need one to become a certified activity director. With a bachelor's degree, you can be certified as the more prestigious-sounding recreational therapist. My experience is that most activity departments in nursing homes have directors with less than a four-year degree. People with bachelor's degrees—in a manifestation of the law of inverse proportionality—wind up as administrators of recreation in the larger facilities, not actually calling "B twelve" on bingo afternoon but supervising those who do. Most of the camp counselors who watch our precious children don't have college degrees, either. Showing someone a good time is not an academic exercise.

When your cruise director is certified, it means the fun is certified too. There's an element of Kantianism here—showing someone a good time out of duty rather than enjoyment or desire. The fifth of the Ten Commandments says, "Honor thy father and mother." God is commanding us to honor our parents, not to love them. Christianity is a faith-based religion. There are no enumerated duties. It's of our own free will that we accept Jesus as our savior. We are not commanded to love Him. So a Jew could argue that under Christianity it's hit-or-miss whether we take care of our parents. With Judaism, it's because God said so.

All the regulations and certifications that are the backbone of nursing home culture are Kantian too. As a society, we find it unwieldy to simply throw a bunch of old people into a space supervised by younger people without enumerating their duties. I'll admit that my aesthetic sense prefers a less scripted approach. Emotionally, I'd prefer Rodney King's, "Can't we all just get along?" It's preferable when love and duty coincide—when you not only honor your parents but love to do so. But if you can't get the staff to care for you out of love, I'll settle for regulations and commandments.

It's Thursday, November 8, 2007.

"Mrs. Calabash [I've found her, Mr. Durante], what is today's date?"

Mrs. Calabash—weathered face, hand tremor, but still, with penetrating steel-gray eyes—turns to the wall, which gives me a chance to slyly check my watch because I forgot too, and looks at the activity calendar.

"I knew it but I forgot."

To avoid embarrassment, I offer my usual bromide: "It's hard to keep track of the date, what with no newspaper, no checks to write, no appointment book."

I give her credit for knowing enough to look at the calendar.

"It's Thursday, November 8, Mrs. Calabash. I notice they're going to have a birthday party today. Are you going?"

"It's not mine, so why bother? And if it was mine, why bother too?"

I see that Mrs. Calabash has not lost her sense of humor, even as it has turned to the darkside.

The staff is concerned Mrs. Calabash spends all her time in solitary play. But her solitary play has brought her almost to the end of *Her Father's House* by Belva Plain, as I can tell by the bookmark. Belva Plain, born 1919, is the queen of nursing home reading for those who can still read.

"My mother read her," I confide to Mrs. Calabash.

"Oh, she's all right, but I'd rather be going out to dinner with my friends. They're all dead."

The weekly activity calendar from which Mrs. Calabash tried to puzzle out the date is a design feature of every nursing home room, one for every resident posted on the wall by the bed. I look at these calendars and I see no empty spaces. It's as full as Paris Hilton's party schedule.

Here's a list of the activities I found on a typical calendar: exercise, coffee hour, ice cream social, bingo, Mass, Bible ministry, bigband piano nostalgia, crossword puzzles, trivia contest, crafts, beach bag tic-tac-toe, beach ball bowling, movie: *Woman of the Year* with Tracy and Hepburn, needle crafts, flower arrangement, and residents' council.

With all this scheduled fun, how can there be "no observable behavior"?

Many of the residents don't even know there is an activity calendar beside them on the wall, let alone its contents. It would be easy to blame their low awareness on their low mental status, but quick: Do you know how many calories there are in the Big Mac? There's a chart at every McDonald's. What are the side effects of that Lipitor you have been taking? There's an info sheet with every prescription. Most people don't bother with these things.

The research on medical informed consent—all those forms you sign telling you about the risks when you have surgery or get a CAT scan—reveals that the cogent among us don't really know what's going on. Despite mandated informed consent, most studies show patients retain only a limited awareness of medical risks, and they're not even aware of their ignorance. For example, one study from Dublin, "Informed Consent: A Patients' Perspective," surveyed cancer patients about their knowledge of complications after the usual pre-procedure briefing. The results? "More than 80 percent of respondents were happy with the information provided, however, over half of these could not list even one complication of their operation."

Awareness of risks aside, there's similar ignorance about privacy rights. In 1997, the federal government enacted the Health Insurance Portability and Accountability Act (HIPAA). Go into any doctor's office, and they hand you a privacy rights statement and you sign that you understand it. Privacy is as old as medicine, as old as the Hippocratic Oath, which states, in part, "What I may see or hear in the course of the treatment or even outside of the treatment in regard to the life of men, which on no account one must spread abroad, I will keep to myself, holding such things shameful to be spoken about." A modern version by Louis Lasagna in 1964, and sworn to by many newly minted doctors says, "I will respect the privacy of my patients, for their problems are not disclosed to me that the world may know." As a psychologist, I didn't swear to either oath, although I follow a code of ethics that mandates privacy, which predated HIPAA. If we were literal about these things, none of us could write about our patients, and there goes a whole genre. I adhere to the mandate by scrupulously writing about my patients so that not one of them or their families could read this book and know it was about them.

But despite HIPAA, despite all those forms and postings in medical offices, patients retain only a vague awareness of their privacy rights and the extent to which informed consent signs away many of those rights. A typical study, "Patients' Perceptions About the Privacy of Their Medical Records," revealed that "patients were generally unaware, misinformed, or confused about data and personal health information practices and believed that there was less data sharing than is routinely practiced in health care." We can certainly forgive poor Mrs. Calabash for not knowing the date or when bingo begins.

Practically, privacy in a public institution is impossible. They post notices not even to speak out loud the name of a resident— loose lips sink ships. But when I'm looking for a resident's chart, I have to browse through all the other charts on the rack. I'm looking for DeMatteo, but "Hmm, D'Antonio, isn't that my wife's cousin?" is an impossible thought to suppress.

In my private life as a patient, I throw my hands up, live with no expectation of confidentiality, and smile in the camera.

———————

I walk into Sedgmoor Manor, and there's a crowd in the dining room—a room that doubles as the center of activities. This reminds me of my kids' school. It doesn't have a lunchroom, but a multipurpose room. Roll back the tables, unfold the chairs, and let's put on a show. At Sedgmoor, it's two p.m. and it's bowling. Not that there's a bowling alley. When my kids were little they had their own bowling set—all plastic. You set up the pins and hurled the beach ball–size bowling ball. Then you had to set them all up again. Tedious. It's the same with bowling at Sedgmoor. No automatic lanes, the tedium and setting up the pins by hand, but these folks have time on their hands.

Both childhood and old age come with toys that are larger than life. Developing or deteriorating fine motor skills require large objects to hold on to. It's not just the bowling. When they do a crossword puzzle, it's a giant crossword puzzle on a giant poster board. It's the large-print version of not just books but life. Everything is not only big but also loud. I'm happy that even at my age loud still sounds loud—even though I sometimes have to ask my ten-year-old what SpongeBob just confided to Patrick.

In their later years, my parents would blare the TV, but I can remember them telling me as a child to turn it down and move back from the screen because I'd hurt my eyes. My kids do the same, and channeling my parents, I provide the same admonishments. Children don't have failing vision or hearing, but they like to immerse themselves in the experience. In Norman Malcolm's memoir about the childlike philosopher Ludwig Wittgenstein, he wrote that his mentor would always sit in the front row at movies. It blocked everything else out in his busy head.

For Wittgenstein, recreation—what little he had of it—was just recreation. But even Freud said, "A woman is a woman, but a good cigar is a smoke." When we burden play with being the work of childhood, are we robbing it of its playfulness? When we load down recreation with the modifier "therapy," are we taking away the fun? Maybe that's why a resident refuses—particularly a mentally sharp one—to go to recreation. It's too much work, not fun enough.

Most people—particularly most retired people—don't live their lives on a schedule. The nursing home activity calendar is yet another reminder that it's an institution. My kids, typical early-twenty-first-century middle class, have a more scheduled life than I have, or ever had. The music lessons, soccer, baseball, basketball, Hebrew school routine. I'm the proverbial soccer mom chauffeur—driving my kids to all their scheduled, structured activities. They get to hear me go on about my spontaneous childhood—going down to the schoolyard where we kids would choose up sides for basketball. Today, if you don't have a schedule, you don't have a life—and sometimes I feel as if I have no life except to adhere to my children's schedule. My father and many residents with significant dementia refuse recreation. I argued with the staff against his right to refuse recreation. I suggested—human rights advocate that I am—just wheeling him over without asking. My dad's refusal—or "noncompliance," to use the term of art—to go to recreation could have been a vestigial effort to retain control. Just saying no to everything is a kind of mastery—even when it made as little apparent sense as everything else in his cognitively diminished life.

Sharp-minded residents also refuse recreation. They're sitting in their rooms reading *The Hartford Courant*, watching and actually paying attention to TV—or wheeling themselves outside, maybe with a stopover at the day-care center—to sit in the sun. "These people around here. I can't relate to them. You talk to them and get nothing back but nonsense." I hear a fair amount of that too.

I seldom get a complaint from staff or residents when I remove them from an activity to do my psychology thing.

I'll ask the nurse or aide, "I'm looking for Mrs. Kletchner. Could you tell me what she looks like, please?"

"Oh, she's old, in a wheelchair, and white hair."

"That narrows it down."

A little standard-issue nursing home humor.

"I think she's at rec."

This could be bowling. Or it could be the giant crossword puzzle. Or it could be trivia. How did Glenn Miller die? Plane crash? Car crash? Or any of the other pastimes that do little more than pass time.

I walk over to the rec room. Look for someone that looks like staff and ask could I please see Mrs. Kletchner. Typically, she'd be seated at a table in her wheelchair. I'll announce myself. "Hi, I'm Ira Rosofsky. I'm a psychologist, and I just want to chat with you a bit." I may have to say it quite loud, violating HIPAA. A quizzical look from Mrs. Kletchner as the staff member and I rearrange wheelchairs to make a path for wheeling Mrs. Kletchner down the hall.

I'll say, "Sorry to take you away."

"Oh, it doesn't matter. I was just killing time waiting for lunch."

The only activity that sometimes sparks resistance is for bingo. It's the queen of nursing home activities. Maybe it is important because, unlike plastic bowling or big-band trivia, it's not an ersatz nursing home activity but one the people might have gone to before the nursing home. Except here, there aren't hundred-dollar stakes. It's not the church basement with conviviality and a stop at the doughnut shop for more coffee on the way home. Here it's twenty-five cents and nowhere to spend it. Mrs. Salamanca, a ten-year nursing home resident, opened her nightstand drawer and showed me a mess of quarters from years of bingo. But it's the sacred activity, as sacred if not more so than the weekly Mass with the portable altar and cross the traveling priest pulls out of his briefcase, or the Bible study meeting that doesn't get much beyond Jesus Loves You.

My father gained a bit of religiosity at his Jewish nursing home. Jews need ten people for group prayer, a *minyan*—ten males if you're Orthodox. Although they had issues with wheeling him against his supposed will to recreation, there was no problem among his coreligionists with wheeling him to services—a religious obligation—and putting a yarmulke on his head. You don't need to be legally competent in civil society to be counted as an adult man in the Jewish religion. Obeying the Jewish commandments doesn't require intention, just behavior. Your heart doesn't have to be in it, so dementia does not preclude you from the fulfillment of your religious obligations. Dad affected the yarmulke style for a while, went to services daily. There was a big Passover Seder every year, and my family of five joined him at it. I remember him saying over the soup not a blessing but "Needs more salt" as he proceeded to empty half a shaker into it. I'd get two mitzvahs—good deeds that fulfill commandments—for showing up that day: one for being at the Seder, another for honoring my father.

It's the day before Thanksgiving. I'm at Newburn Rehabilitation, meeting with James Rathscroft. Just fifty-three—it's been eight years since his Parkinson's diagnosis. He has only a slight hand tremor as he sits in his wheelchair, required because of frequent falls and general weakness. He has a youthful, soft look. Big doe eyes, pudgy—no doubt aided by his wheelchair inactivity—but he has powerful forearms from all that pushing of the wheels over the years. He didn't have a WanderGuard, because he had agreed to a seat belt, which also gives him the frequent opportunity to unfasten it, stand up, walk around, and get yelled at by nurses and aides. His mind puzzles the staff—dementia or delusions?

"What's today's date?"

"November 21, 2007."

Perfect on this, and all the mental status questions—the date, the day, the place, the president, his mother's maiden name, spelling "world" backward. He aces it.

"How long have you been here?"

"A few months. I'm just going to get my strength back, and get back home."

Rathscroft has been at Newburn for almost two years, so I'm trying to differentiate between whether it's a psychotic delusion or a neurotic denial.

"Is your family coming tomorrow to visit for Thanksgiving?"

"No, I'm going home tomorrow."

Afterward, I mentioned to the nurse that he's expecting to go home. She confirmed that at the young age of fifty-three, this is his permanent home.

"We talk about it. He comes to the care planning meetings where we remind him, but he doesn't either remember or believe it."

I ask if he's confused about maybe going home just for Thanksgiving.

"I don't think he's on the list. But you never know, sometimes the family shows up without telling us."

Thanksgiving, Christmas, and the Fourth of July are three days when many people—with elaborate preparation—go home. For a lucky few, the nursing home takes on aspects of an adult boarding school.

Most of the time you're a member of the Dead Poets Society, but on holidays you might be a family member. Some people have more connections to their families than only on holidays—doing lunch with a daughter, home for Sunday football with a son. These might be residents who don't appear to need the 24/7 of nursing home, if only they wouldn't be in danger of leaving the tub running, flooding the house, or worse, forgetting about the stove and burning down the house. They might have kids who are working or don't want the responsibility of around-the-clock caregiving. They might be unable to afford assisted living. They hang their hats at the nursing home but walk unassisted to the car with the kid taking them to the hot dog shack by the shore.

I've heard, "Mom's at the nursing home, but we take her out all the time."

We took my father on field trips, even after he had broken two hips and was mostly in the wheelchair. The head of the physical therapy department trained me how to do it. Wheel him out to the car, lock the wheelchair, stand up Dad, one person on each side as he turns and backs into the car seat, gripping his walker. Reverse the procedure at my house, except here he has to walk up the five steps to my front door. Linda's on one side, I'm on the other with a grip on his belt in the back, spotting him so he won't topple back down the stairs. Quite a production. All these mitzvahs filling books of green stamps for a heaven I don't believe in.

So it's mostly me visiting Dad. When I'm at work in the area, I drop by for lunch and buy a chocolate-chip cookie at the bakeshop as a peace offering when he says, "Get the hell out of here!" I bring my youngest son, who is not in school. A math prodigy at the age of four, he's an expert at pushing "3" on the elevator. If there still were jobs for elevator operators, I joke to passengers, he'd have all the skills. Sometimes I drop by with a book and sit in Dad's room with him. He has large-print *Reader's Digest*s, and the staff says he's reading. Maybe, but I never see it.

Singing appears to be one of the last things of normal life to go. Stutterers gain fluency with singing. People with dementia stare blankly or erupt irrationally at bingo, but music taps into deeply laden pathways. Songs like "Home on the Range" or "Bicycle Built for Two" remain earworms stuck in the minds of the most addled. My father, joyless in many ways—he once told me in his cogent days that it's hard for him to smile—would pace around our family apartment singing his songs, not a bad voice. We call them standards today—"Fly Me to the Moon," "Love Is a Many Splendored Thing." He could hit the high notes and the fortes. I enjoy going to the sing-alongs at the nursing home, a short wheelchair push into the dining room. He's there before he can object. The activity worker is comely, plays the guitar, and I tap my feet right along.

I buy him a CD player along with Frank Sinatra, Dean Martin, and Perry Como albums. That is, until the player disappears, likely stolen by the staff. Occasionally, I'll put on "Catch a Falling Star" and think of Dad and Mom still together. It's a childhood memory. *The Perry Como Show*. Something my parents could agree about. In harmony. Except for me. I want Jackie Gleason.

On the weekend, my whole family shows up, and we wheel him into the courtyard. Chocolate-chip cookies for not just Dad but the kids. We sit in the sun, and there are other families. Some smokers in the corner. As the shadows shift, we follow the sun. We're a tableau. Could be Seurat. *Sunday Afternoon in the Courtyard with Dad*.

Despite honoring my father, I experience episodes of guilt when I see the involvement of others. Some residents require no recreation schedule, no psychiatric intervention, no bingo. As I've said, if Mom can't be home, we'll bring home to Mom. On more than one occasion, it's the child who never got married and who lived at home with Mom. Spending long hours with Mom at the nursing home is only a change of location. When Mom dies, many of these unmarried children caretakers don't know what to do with themselves. Others feel liberated—an adult after all those decades of providing care yet remaining a child to the parent.

Experiencing these manifold types of domesticity leads me to a more expansive view of civil unions than the garden-variety gay activist. Why restrict the expansion of civil union—or marriage—to only gays and lesbians? What about all the siblings and parents and children who have lived together for decades? Shouldn't the unions of the proverbial maiden aunts have rights and recognition too?

I'm sitting at the nursing station at Neville's Cross. There's a large alcove by a window with massed wheelchairs facing a large corkboard on wheels on which are tacked about twenty 8-by-11-inch sheets of paper. At the board is a woman who might be a recreational therapist, an activity director, or a mere recreational worker. Doesn't matter. I'm in a hurry to get home, so I'm concentrating on my notes, and catch only a few minutes of the game of concentration. The rec lady turns over one of the sheets.

"Number twelve. It's a butterfly. Does anyone remember where the other butterfly is?"

Blank stares mostly.

Finally, someone pipes up. "Number seventy-five."

"Oh, that's a good guess, Sophie, but there is no seventy-five."

For some reason, the scene reminds me of one from *Blackboard Jungle*, when Mr. Edwards attempts to engage his hoodlum students by playing his precious 78-rpm jazz records. The students' indifference turns to unrestrained adolescent rage as they first smash the records, and then Mr. Edwards himself. At the nursing home, rage is labeled as dementia with behavioral disturbance and treated with Zyprexa or Depakote.

I can only imagine what it is like to be in the mind of a person with dementia, but William James comes to mind. The brother of Henry, William was the founder of the pragmatist school of philosophy, a father of scientific psychology, and a noted doggerel poet: "Hoggamus, higgamus, men are polygamous. Higgamus, hoggamus, women monogamous." This revelation is reputed to have emerged from one of his many enjoyable nitrous oxide highs—"I strongly urge others to repeat the experiment, which with pure gas is short and harmless enough." He believed the laughing-gas buzz provided "intense metaphysical illumination." Getting high not only helped James understand for the first time the philosopher Georg Wilhelm Friedrich Hegel—much tougher than Kant—but inspired his theory that drugs were the original basis of all religious experience. James's epiphany predated by almost a century the injunction of another Harvard psychology professor, Timothy Leary, to "Turn on, tune in, and drop out."

Although he experimented with drugs, as a psychologist William James was more theoretical than experimental. He originated the counterintuitive cognitive theory of emotion. Naïvely, we believe we see the bear, he scares us, we run. James countered that we see the bear, we automatically run, then we name the reaction: fear. The sight of the bear causes all animals smaller than the bear to tremble, pump out adrenaline, and run. Humans can put a name on the automatic reaction and call it emotion. In this sense, James was the father of cognitive behavioral therapy, which holds, in part, that emotional dysfunction arises out of mislabeling experience—failure labeled as helplessness rather than as instructive.

I could work up a phenomenological theory of dementia here. James wrote that for a baby the world is "one great blooming, buzzing confusion." He was actually wrong on this point. As anyone who took introductory psychology ought to remember, an experiment by Robert Fantz in 1961 showed that the perceptual world of a newborn is quite a bit more organized than James imagined. In a clever experiment, Fantz presented two pictures to babies. One had a human face, the other a bull's-eye. The babies spent twice as much time looking at the face as the bull's-eye. This suggests that the baby's mind, rather than the tabula rasa—the blank slate—made famous by the philosopher John Locke and apparently seconded by James, is prewired to organize experience into recognizable categories. Babies are quite Kantian in their outlook. In his *Critique of Pure Reason,* Kant argued that experience is not purely empirical, but that we bring a priori (before experience) templates to organize our perception of the world. The person with dementia has misplaced the templates with which we organize our experience; he has lost the ability to name his experiences. It's not for the baby but for my father that the world is blooming, buzzing confusion.

So the game of concentration at Neville's Cross is just one part of the bloom and the buzz. There is only a diminished I, a shattered ego, to make sense of it all. People with dementia appear to have no boundaries between what's going on inside their heads and outside their heads. Engaging residents in a group setting is a challenge. It's like talking to someone learning to speak English. Sitting face-to-face, focusing on the interaction, you can communicate. But take her to lunch with your friends and she's lost in the flow of casual conversation. Until close to the end, I could sit with my father in a quiet room and make some reasonable verbal contact.

"Would you like another cookie, Dad?"

"Yes."

A recreational activity is only one of many stimuli competing for increasingly limited attention. To engage the confused, you need close to one-to-one, would-you-like-another-cookie relationships. Families who can arrange to spend hours with Mom or Dad provide the best activity programs. There are no activity calendars necessary for these off-the-cuff family recreation programs. Companionably sitting with Mom or Dad, watching some TV, wheeling them outside, wiping the dribble off the chin, and saying "Hello in there" is more than enough— and you could bring your laptop and get a lot of work done. One-to-one is well beyond the means or desires of our current system—even as the young disabled get personal assistants to get them through the day at school. But I can dream about an hour a day where everybody—the administrators, the CNAs, the nurses, the office workers, the kitchen staff, the podiatrist, and me too would have to sit with a resident and just hold a hand. That could do some good.

Mrs. Horowitz, sound of mind, frail of body, likes to read.

"They say you're not going to any of the activities, Mrs. Horowitz."

On the table in front of her is Sue Grafton. It's *S is for Silence*— an appropriate title for the reclusive Mrs. Horowitz. The bookmark is near the end.

"I have nothing in common with those people. When I'm not feeling sorry for myself, I feel sorry for them. Being with them makes me worry that I'm going to be like them."

"Do you go to any of the activities?"

"The only activity I'd like would be to be able to get out of this chair and walk, so I could walk out of here."

"I see you haven't lost your sense of humor, Mrs. Horowitz."

Mrs. Horowitz, despite being in the nursing home, retains her sense of autonomy, a sense of self—making her own pleasures as best she can. Then, when they notice, they worry she's reclusive.

There are many Mrs. Horowitzes in nursing homes, perfectly cogent and no more depressed than anyone else who traded a home of fifty years for a nursing home. She's arguably unsafe at home, but sharp enough to see beyond bingo in the nursing home. Look at her nodding off in her wheelchair and you may observe "no observable behavior." But who wouldn't prefer a nap to returning to the office after lunch? When she wakes up from her nap, she could read a book, do her crosswords, watch *Jeopardy!* and solve her own trivia. Scattered around the places I go, I see a beachhead of computers here and there. When my boomer generation hits these shores, we'll demand Wi-Fi. My thirteen-year-old daughter can sit at the computer for hours instant-messaging her friends while they all check out a cute skirt on the American Eagle website. She's reclusive enough now. Imagine her a century from now in whatever the nursing home has become.

Mrs. Horowitz just wants to read.

Assisted-living centers are the halfway home between home and the nursing home. You could think of them as a reverse purgatory between the heaven of independence and the hell of total dependence.

Many of the people I meet in nursing homes, if not a majority, could be in assisted-living homes—if they could afford it. They need someone to organize their medication, help them take a bath, get in or out of bed, or remind them to use their walker. Few people need the intensive care of a nursing home.

It's a serious irrationality of our health care system that we are much more willing to pay for the cure than the prevention. In my outpatient psychotherapy days, I would have to approach insurance companies on bended knee to ask for more than six measly weeks of psychotherapy. When they failed to authorize more time, I'd think they're saying, "We ain't gonna pay for no twenty-five years of Woody Allen psychoanalysis." But what if the patient who is denied more outpatient therapy tries to kill himself and winds up in the hospital?

The denied additional psychotherapy sessions would have cost a few hundred dollars. The hospital stay could run into tens of thousands. The denied outpatient therapy might have prevented the hospitalization. Where's the logic in that?

Outpatient psychotherapy is to psychiatric hospitalization as assisted-living centers are to nursing homes.

The average annual cost of an assisted-living center is $35,000; the average nursing home costs $75,000. Some can afford to pay the assisted-living costs out-of-pocket indefinitely. But if you live long enough, the money will run out, and you will need to go on the government dole. Medicaid will not pay for assisted living, but will gladly pay more than twice as much for the nursing home. The gold standard for care is to provide it in the least restrictive environment, but in the case of the elderly the payment goes toward the most restrictive environment.

There are approximately 500,000 residents in the 33,000 assisted-living facilities in the United States. Their average age is eighty-five—equivalent to the average age of people in nursing homes. Four-fifths are female. The differences between a typical assisted-living facility and a nursing home are both obvious and subtle. An assisted-living center looks more like an upscale college dormitory than a hospital. You get an apartment rather than a hospital room. The apartment is missing a full kitchen. There's only a sink, a fridge, and a microwave, as in many motel rooms. They usually serve only one meal per day in the dining room, so the microwave comes in handy for reheating leftovers. The apartment has safety features—pull-cords to alert the staff, grab handles in the bathroom. When you're relatively spry and young, you might not want more from assisted living than the roof over your head plus the meals. You might still be driving—which also makes you as popular among your peers as a teenager with a car. You're going out to movies, shopping, or popping in on your kids. You just don't have to maintain your big house anymore. As your needs for assistance increase, the costs are added on to the basic $35,000 for room and board. Need an aide to get you dressed, dole out your meds, help you bathe? That will be at least fifteen dollars per hour. As it adds up, your family might think it would be cheaper for you to run through your money and go on Medicaid in the nursing home. Or you might slip and fall or get sick, which will also provide you with a pathway to the nursing home. If your money doesn't run out or you don't break anything, but your mind starts slipping, they might transfer you to the assisted-living facility's dementia unit—more intensive staff contact, locked exits, and a more focused activity schedule. But before you reach the dementia unit, you might be in a facility with tony activities—lectures rather than trivia, chamber music rather than "Down by the Old Mill Stream," exercises in the pool, movie night in the theater followed by cucumber finger sandwiches reminiscent of your teas at Smith College sixty years ago—even a sip of sherry.

Pervading this, though, is a sense of *No Exit* even if you're not in the locked dementia unit. Your only foreseeable options for the future are death or a deeper level of institutionalization including a move to a nursing home.

"It's just like high school," an assisted-living social worker young enough to have had a recent recollection of high school told me.

In the world of *The Sopranos*, the dutiful sons sent their mothers to the upscale Green Grove Retirement Community. David Chase got the name right, Green Grove rather than Autumn Leaves. Paulie "Walnuts" Gualtieri is proud to be able to afford the monthly $4,000 for his mother, Nucci. But her friends are shunning her. Talking to his mother's friends does no good, so he, a man of action, breaks the arm of one of the ladies' sons and Mom gets to sit with the cool kids.

Paulie Walnuts aside, there is a sorting out of who sits where in the dining room, who gets invited to drinks before dinner, and who replaces the just-deceased member of the bridge foursome. The more competent want to surround themselves with their peers. The frailer minds and body are unwelcome omens of the probable future.

There's a natural sorting out, as in high school. Not in terms of the popular kids, the jocks, the hippies, the goths, and the nerds, but a more callous sorting out in terms of cognitive capacity. If you are not capable of holding up your end of the conversation, you're not going to be invited to a table where there is a conversation. Nucci Gualtieri lagged a few steps behind the others, and they tried to cut her out of the herd.

At the Roarkes' Drift Retirement Community, I meet Mrs. Rita MacKenzie. It's a medium-grade assisted-living center. The couches in the common area are fabric, not leather. The carpet could be thicker. I hear a hollow thud from the cheap construction materials as my big frame walks down the corridors to the MacKenzie apartment. Each apartment has some pictures by the door. I pass a photo of the Verrazano-Narrows Bridge, a model sailing ship, the rocky coast of Maine, a resident's photo along with grandchildren and great-grandchildren. At Mrs. MacKenzie's door is a photo of what I learn are the Canadian Rockies, and there's also a little display shelf with a replica of the Eiffel Tower.

They tell me Mrs. MacKenzie won't leave her room. Her meals are brought in from the dining room by her aide, who helps her get up, eat lunch, and get back to bed. In her room are the usual remains of a long life. Photos, bric-a-brac, oil portraits, vintage furniture, and stacks of correspondence and magazines. Very few books.

Mrs. MacKenzie is as tiny as a child. If she told me she was in her seventies, I wouldn't blink. Blue, mostly clear eyes, with only a tinge of red, and wetness along the lower eyelid. Skin remarkably unlined for any woman over the age of sixty.

"How old are you, Mrs. MacKenzie?" It's one of my standard mental status questions.

"I'm going to be one hundred four on Saturday. I was born July 14, 1903."

"Bastille Day, eh?"

She appreciates the "eh," being Canadian, born in Saskatoon, Saskatchewan. I love that exotic, alliterating name, but shiver internally knowing that it gets to many degrees below zero, global warming or no.

Innocently I ask, "You have any memories of World War One?"

I'm making conversation, but her eyes get wetter.

"I remember my brother Bobby, only seventeen—I used to ride on his shoulders—marching off to war. He looked so fine. Three months later, he was killed at the Somme. Every day I think about him. I said I'd never forget. The Eiffel Tower is from when I went to visit his grave."

Bobby is more than a lifetime away—ninety-three years away. She was a girl when he left, and he died at an age young enough to be one of her great-grandchildren today. Rita Clarkson went on to marry Tom MacKenzie, an oil engineer.

"We traveled all over the world, until we settled in New York when Tom got a job in the home office."

"How did you wind up in Connecticut?"

"Well, Tom died more than twenty years ago, and I was already eighty, so my son, who had moved up to Connecticut, got worried about me being alone. I sold my home in Rye and moved into a condo near my son."

Her son is seventy-seven, which doesn't quite attain the filial agedness of the one-hundred-two-year-old mother and her eighty-two-year-old daughter I met at another facility. They were both in bad shape, but Tom MacKenzie, Jr., his mom tells me, is currently visiting his daughter in Italy, and she's upset she can't be with them.

The staff tells me she's depressed, a woman who was living on her own just six months ago. I ask her how she passes her time. Does she like to read?

"Oh, I never was much of a reader. More of an active person. I liked to travel. And I like my TV shows."

"They tell me you don't go to any of the activities. That you prefer to stay by yourself."

"Wouldn't you? Who wants to be with a bunch of old hags! Half of them just sit around and gossip. The other half don't know their ass from their elbow."

She sees my expression. "At my age, I say want I want." And then she laughs.

"And there's this fellow who is always trying to flirt with me—a mere child of eighty-seven. He should be ashamed."

This from someone who was already nine years old when the *Titanic* sank, whose brother disappeared at the Battle of the Somme, whose childhood friends perished in the great postwar flu epidemic, who had her first child before the 1929 stock market crash. She finds it hard to reconcile her ancient status with her sense of self.

"I'm still me, unless I feel the aching in my bones or look at my walker."

Me too. I can still feel as immature as ever, and when I look into the mirror I wonder, "Who is that guy?" I have a feeling that Mrs. MacKenzie avoids the mirrors in her apartment too.

Mrs. MacKenzie has it all going on except any kind of reasonable life expectancy. In the purgatory of assisted living, everything is subtraction. It's a high school where graduation is only a negative thing—death or the nursing home. This is the underlying current, the insistent minor-key bass line walking below every illusory melody of independence. Even as they call one class of residents independent living.

Mrs. MacKenzie complained about her would-be flirting beau, which raises the question of vice and pleasure. There's still plenty of sex and drugs among the aged, even if not rock and roll.

As children, there's the "ick" factor when we think about our parents doing it, let alone our grandparents. But grandparents and great-grandparents do it—and academics confirm it. A group at the University of Chicago's National Opinion Research Center (NORC) recently surveyed the sexual behavior of 3,005 elderly adults.

The survey—"A Study of Sexuality and Health Among Older Adults in the United States," published August 2007 in *The New England Journal of Medicine*—confirms that old people are making a lot of whoopee, often as much as people many years younger: "In our study, the frequency of sexual activity reported by respondents who were sexually active was similar to that reported among adults 18 to 59 in the 1992 National Health and Social Life Survey." A majority of both men and women fifty-five to seventy-five who are in a relationship are having sex at least twice each month. Men have a better time of it. They desire it more than women. And, being scarce, it is easier for them to find a mate.

For single elderly people, there's less action—as at any age. Only 22 percent of single men, and 4 percent of single women are sexually active. But masturbation remains the lonely person's friend—as well as an auxiliary means of pleasure for the married. More than half of the men and a quarter of the women surveyed rely on it regularly.

So we remain human to the end. Poor health—not age—puts an end to the fun and frolic. Male health problems are the number-one reason for the end of sex. And beware the end of desire. It could mean the end of life. One of the researchers, Edward Lauman, cautioned that sexual inactivity is an important marker of poor health. Doctors should be sure to ask about it. "When sexual health begins to deteriorate, it is an important warning sign of more profound health problems."

I am sure that independent residents in assisted-living centers remain as sexually active as those surveyed by NORC. A gent, old enough to be my father, dispensed with my services along with bragging about his fifty-eight-year-old girlfriend—young enough to be his daughter. Psychotherapy remains at any age a poor substitute for the scent of a woman. But in nursing homes and among more dependent folks in assisted living, the only notice I get of sexual activity is when the staff refers to an old codger groping the nurses, or the guy who was found in the bed of a confused and helpless woman, or the one masturbating in front of the aides. I've never seen a Viagra prescription in a nursing home chart—although its use is otherwise prevalent among our elders.

Sex in the nursing home is more of a problem than a pleasure. Dementia breaks down inhibition. All your life you may have wanted to, but you confined yourself to coveting. Now the reins are off. In my grad student days, back when there was a rash of airplane hijackers, I evaluated one who confided, "I was driving by the airport and saw the sign 'Delta is ready when you are.'" So when you hear inside your confused head, "Reach out and touch somebody," the voice could be your libido unbound and not a remembrance of some old phone company jingle.

That's not to say there are no intimate relationships among those with dementia. Sandra Day O'Connor's husband with Alzheimer's had a handholding girlfriend. I've seen solicitous beaus pushing their more disabled girlfriends around in wheelchairs. I've seen young people with paraplegia or multiple sclerosis or Parkinson's proudly indicate the photos of their significant others. But that's about as far as it can go for these confined people who retain the same sexual desires as you or me. It is about as hard to find privacy when you are living in one of these public places as it is for teenagers living under their parents' roofs—probably harder. There is a sprinkling of spouses sharing nursing home rooms. But their doors are always open too. Even though many residents act as if they are in a hotel, there are no "Do Not Disturb" signs. Prisons have a more liberal version of conjugal visits.

We could chalk up the absence of sex in nursing homes to poor heath and frailty. But I'd like to move beyond bingo, to utter the word "sex" in a nursing home without modifying it with "harassment" or "offense." It's arguably illegal to prohibit sexual activity in the nursing home. OBRA commands facilities to "support residents in preferred activity," and it established a bill of rights that includes the right to privacy; the right to the accommodation of medical, physical, psychological, and social needs; the right to be treated with dignity; and the right to self-determination. How could privacy, dignity, meeting one's personal needs, and self-determination not add up to sex? Do we have to wait until my iconoclastic boomer generation shows up to make a major stink out of this?

Among the retarded citizens community, there is an ongoing conversation about sexuality—about the tricky balance between sexual rights and sexual exploitation. Most adults in nursing homes—unlike many retarded persons—are legally competent. Old age and sex are not oil and water.

I'll admit it could lead to some intriguing new job responsibilities for the activity director. Tuesday at three: Viagra versus Cialis versus Levitra. Wednesday at ten: Sex toys for the single octogenarian.

Sex aside, it's hard to get a drink. There's Sean Hanrahan and his celebratory Red Sox beer and few others.

For most of the residents, Prohibition was a story they heard from their parents—as my cousins and I heard about our fathers' adventures in World War II. During the Depression, alcohol was a legal part of their often grim lives. They experienced postwar society with the cocktail dress and the cocktail party. This is another part of life they leave behind. There's abundant evidence that moderate drinking is good for you. But, curiously, in the few institutions where you can get a drink, you need a doctor's prescription. It's a drug among drugs, not a beverage.

I know that alcohol abuse among the elderly is the "invisible epidemic." I know that the cocktails before dinner at assisted-living centers could be a continuation of a lifetime of excess. I know I see some folks with liver cirrhosis and others with alcohol-induced dementia and still others with both. But, in nursing homes, our elders have entered a new age of Prohibition—one more infantilization. No doubt a doctor would say, "I have to be careful with alcohol because of all the other drugs they're taking"—without any sense of irony.

But tobacco, that most dangerous drug is rampantly not prohibited.

Nursing homes often call themselves "health centers," yet they are last-gasp holdouts of the cigarette. The smokers are mostly old and mostly poor. They're the welfare folks with $54 monthly wheeling-around money—that is, after the state kicks in $75,000 for room and board.

At five bucks a pack, they have the kind of life where you choose between smokes or a haircut. We are not quite in Marlboro Country, but in a place where the Greatest Generation can show the flag with a cheap brand of generics called USA.

Tightly controlled, the cigarettes are locked away except for the three or four daily outdoor breaks, two smokes per break. Johnny B. Goode can't walk around with his pack under his T-shirt sleeve as he did fifty years ago, in the fifties. Johnny, who wouldn't remember where he put them, is not a good risk for matches.

When I show up to do my psychotherapy thing and Johnny's smoking, it's hard to see him—harder than when he's eating or at bingo.

It is sacred time, in all kinds of weather. Perversely, it's Johnny's only time for fresh air and the great outdoors. Over the PA, I hear,

"All smokers meet at the nursing station," and that lights the smoking lamp—a ritual tucked between medication and moving the bowels. Outside, in the courtyard, an aide, also smoking, sits beside a cabinet from which she dispenses the cigarettes one by one as the wheelchairs roll by.

The staff lamely jokes you can't tell a ninety-year-old the habit could kill him.

For Gary Bonquist, smoking is a way of life. Only forty-three, he always wanted to kill himself. Showing bad judgment, he threw himself out of only the second floor—just enough for morbidity, not enough for mortality. Packed off to the nursing home, his body, now twisted in directions not part of God's original plan, spends its days in one of those recumbent wheelchairs. His family is way off somewhere and not at all interested. He smiles and tells me, "Smoking is my hobby." Whenever I see him he asks, "Have any cigarettes?" I've told him many times I gave it up years ago. But this week he has his pack, and sitting together in the light rain, watching Gary smoke is the only way to have a session. For Gary, it's an extra smoking break. He's an athlete of smoking. It's hard to put the words "athlete" and "smoking" in the same sentence, but Gary pulls it off. If Philip Morris had a championship of smoking, Gary would be world class. I watch the glowing tip of his cigarette race to his lips as he inhales long and deeply. I remember smoke knifing through my lungs, and how I loved it too. Some people have a need to cut themselves. They are numb and they want to feel something, anything. A sharp blade firmly along the forearm is just the thing. Smoking does that on the inside. I'm already lighting Gary's second as he continues to inhale all that life has left for him.

Something in me enjoys smokers crowding around hospital entrances; the image of folks wheeling out their IV stands, sitting in their wheelchairs or unhooking their oxygen to light up. All the patients joined by staff in hospital whites and pinks and greens. An intrepid soul with laryngeal carcinoma might put her cigarette right through the trach tube in her throat. Oh, we few, we happy few, we band of brothers!

Some hospitals have banned the smokers from the entrances. That just kicks the spectacle down the street. Junkies joke that nicotine is much the harder drug to quit. Reformed though I am, I can feel in my gut why POWs traded food dearly for tobacco. AA meetings are dens of caffeine and nicotine—everyone still addicted to something.

When I was a young student, the psych wards had electric cigarette lighters bolted to the wall so the mentally ill could light up while denying them the matches they might otherwise use to light up the whole building.

That's before it was all banned—when ashtrays went from being an industry to becoming collectibles. Curiosities on *Antiques Roadshow*.

Nowadays, if you are in a locked ward, you are out of luck. No smoke for you, say the smoke Nazis. But nursing homes do not ban smoking. At least in this, the old folks know their rights.

I'm just old enough to remember spaceship Earth as a smoke-filled room.

I got my habit bumming smokes in the back rows of college classes. It was a world in which the professor might pause to ask for a light. A pause that refreshed. It was front-page news the day the philosophy department at City College banned smoking soon after the Surgeon General's Report. What a spoilsport. It all began to change.

But look at film from the black-and-white Eisenhower years.

When they're not talking, they're inhaling. (They're all wearing hats too.) I quit many years ago, but I can still miss it, having post-traumatic flashes on how great it would be to light up right now. A heavenly duet with my coffee, I'd draw long, contemplative, perfectly posed drags into my lungs and exhale clouds of smoke across the room as I wonder how to revise this sentence. I smoked unfiltered Camels—I don't need no stinking filters—and loved the lingering smell on my fingers. Lips puckered just so, I could blow some rings. I might even get up and pace around the room, walking a mile with my Camel, waving my arms, scattering ashes, overflowing ashtrays, with the dog off the couch trailing behind me, hours before the wife gets home and says, Look at the mess. Oh lovely mess! I can dream. More likely, I'll go downstairs and do hamster circles on my middle-age-appropriate elliptical machine in front of the TV, green tea in the cup holder, whole grain in my brain.

I do miss it, though, the smoking. Very much the way you miss a lover not good for you but great in bed.

6

YOUNG GIRLS IN
SHORT SKIRTS

Health Care for the Frail and Old

Occasionally, I get to tag along to my company's medical staff meeting. There's a benefit to this. After the meeting, we retire to a wonderful restaurant. This is not at the largesse of my firm, but of one of the several drug companies eager to funnel their wares into our nursing homes. I shake hands with recently minted college graduates dressed for success. They're a couple. Could be the homecoming king and queen. He's better-looking than I could ever be, or want to be. She could be the captain of the cheerleading squad, which she probably is. *The New York Times* documented the cheerleader–drug rep connection. The drug companies deny it's the looks, protesting it's their peppy personalities. Whatever it is, they're the cool kids, the popular ones who wouldn't have let us nerds sit at their table in high school. Now they're happy to feed us pigs at their trough. They're making more money than some of the docs, easily more money than me. Many of them have irrelevant college degrees. Kentucky tried to pass a law requiring science degrees for drug reps, and failed.

Over salad, Ken and Barbie introduce a prominent psychiatrist, also in the employ of Forest Laboratories, who speaks on the wonders of Namenda—only the second drug approved by the FDA for the treatment of Alzheimer's. Prominent psychiatrist is projecting a graph on a screen showing the effects of adding Namenda to Aricept—the first drug in the history of the universe approved for the treatment of Alzheimer's. I don't know many things, but I do know how to read a graph and I'm not impressed. It's bad enough that the Aricept alone doesn't do much to halt the march of dementia. When you add Namenda the march goes on as before. I don't care. I don't care that I'm not a doctor and miss out on the seminars in the Caribbean. I'm eating prime rib, and my gaze shifts to the young girl drug rep in the very short skirt. She's shaking her head in assent as she beams proudly at prominent psychiatrist and his shaky charts.

Some cranky doctors, maybe the ones who didn't get the invite to the Caribbean, resent these peppy, perky reps pulling in six figures without the benefit of years of medical school and years more of debt. Cranky old *JAMA*—*Journal of the American Medical Association*—published an article calling on the pharmaceutical industry, Big Pharma, to commit to some kind of minimal ethical standards in pushing their drugs on doctors. Good luck. In 2000, Big Pharma spent $15.7 billion on wooing doctors—several billion more than they spent on research and development, more even than they spent on advertising to consumers.

Everywhere I go, I see tokens of the drug companies—Zoloft pens, Lipitor Post-it notes, Aricept tote bags. If the drug companies could get away with it, I'm sure they would trick out medical uniforms the way the suits of NASCAR drivers are arrayed with alcohol, tobacco, and lube logos. We are long past our annoyance with stadiums named for beer, telephone companies, banks, and the embarrassingly named Enron Field. I'm surprised that a drug company hasn't joined the naming-rights trend—Eli Manning throwing miracle passes in Eli Lilly field.

Drugs for dementia are a multibillion-dollar part of a $400 billion-a-year worldwide pharmaceutical industry. The dementia segment will grow as we boomers trade in Viagra and Cialis for Aricept and Namenda—despite the shaky lines at the steakhouse presentation. These drugs demonstrate statistically significant effects, which sure sounds good in advertising and on the lips of young girls and hired-gun doctors, but significance is overrated. Suppose you could invent a drug that would enable my extremely nearsighted wife to read the big giant letter on top of the eye chart without her glasses, but none of the smaller letters. Her eyesight would be significantly enhanced, yet—although she is a significantly better driver than I am—I'd still refuse to ride with her without her glasses.

Aricept, approved by the FDA in 1997, has annual sales of $2.3 billion. More than 3.5 million people have taken it. Two-thirds of the revenues come from U.S. prescriptions—a result no doubt of both our affluence and the peculiar nature of our privatized health care system.

Alzheimer's dementia, to the extent we understand it, involves reduced production of the neurotransmitter acetylcholine. Neurotransmitters are chemicals in the brain that facilitate communication among nerve cells. There remains a fair amount of controversy about whether reduced acetylcholine is the cause of Alzheimer's, but Aricept appears to slow its loss.

If you go to the Aricept website, the claims for its effectiveness are somewhat sketchy: "Compared with the placebo group, the typical patient who took Aricept showed improvement on the ADAS-cog test, which measures how well they think, remember, communicate, and figure things out."

How much improvement? They don't say.

I'll say it's very modest. Jacqueline Birks (Oxford University) reviewed thirteen studies involving more than six thousand patients taking Aricept and two similar drugs, Razadyne and Exelon, only to find that drug takers showed, on average, less than three points improvement on a seventy-item mental status exam. That's about a 4 percent difference. Extrapolating this to decline over time—and it's probably not strictly kosher to do this—Aricept will slow your descent into dementia by about fourteen days each year.

What happens when you add Namenda?

Namenda works on another neurotransmitter, glutamate, believed to be associated with memory and learning. If you go to the Namenda website, you will find effectiveness claims startlingly similar to the vague ones for Aricept. Under a bold heading, "Proven Benefits": "People taking Namenda experienced a slower rate of decline in thinking over time."

When I peeked behind that curtain, I found a whole cast of studies that use the "statistically significant" locution. Digging a bit deeper I find a study—the one on which the FDA based its Namenda approval—yielding a range of one to three points difference on a wide-ranging measure of activities of daily living.

Back to our eye-chart analogy, you still wouldn't want to let someone drive without glasses who showed that little visual improvement. And the FDA, in its press release about its approval of Namenda noted, "Although memantine helps treat the symptoms of Alzheimer's disease in some patients, there is no evidence that it modifies the underlying pathology of the disease." In other words, it's a Band-Aid.

This is big business, though. We'll be happy to sell you Band-Aids as long as you keep buying them. Namenda has Pfizer, the developer of Aricept, running scared. In one of its financial advisories, the company cautioned investors: "If this drug [Namenda] is effective there will be no demand for the…Pfizer drug Aricept." And some of the Pfizer young girls in short skirts will be cut off at the knees with the survivors switched to hawking Lipitor, the anticholesterol drug I ingest every day.

It took a country with socialized medicine, a kingdom, to see that the emperor and empress of Alzheimer's meds—Aricept and Namenda—if not naked, are wearing only threadbare clothes.

The UK's National Institute for Health and Clinical Excellence (NICE), akin to our FDA, advises the British National Health Service about the cost effectiveness and permissible uses of drugs— in effect, whether to pay the bill. In September 2007, it issued a tepid damning-with-faint-praise assessment of the uses of Aricept and Namenda. It sanctioned the use of Aricept only for moderate dementia—you remember your name and recognize your wife but forget where you live and who is the queen. Primary care Dr. Welby can't prescribe it either—only geriatric and dementia specialists. If you develop severe dementia—you forget your own name and stare blankly or scream all day—Aricept should be discontinued. And the manufacturer of Namenda won't be buying my British colleagues any steak-and-kidney pies. (Do the Brits have cheerleaders?) Namenda is banished from the formulary—its use forbidden "except as a part of well designed clinical trials."

The NICE doesn't refer to it, but I'd be surprised if it hadn't cast an eye on a University of Birmingham review of Aricept that goes even further. Professor William Gray, director of Birmingham's Clinical Trial Unit, studied 565 noninstitutionalized patients with mild to moderate Alzheimer's. Half took Aricept, half a placebo. Did Aricept delay the progress of the disease or the need for institutional care?

"We've known for some time that patients do better on tests of mental ability when they take these drugs but the improvements were small and we wanted to find out whether patients got benefits that really mattered to them—for example, could they go for a walk and find their way home. In particular, we wanted to know whether people taking donepezil [Aricept] could live at home for longer. If so, this alone would make the drugs worth paying for."

Although the drug did improve mental functioning—"at disappointingly small levels"—it did not delay institutionalization or the progression of dementia. And there were no significant differences in mood, behavior, well-being of caregivers, or costs of caring.

Professor Gray could have been thinking of my eye-chart analogy when he said: "The effects on memory are statistically definite but small. One description is being able to name eleven fruit in a minute instead of ten. Scores on tests of functional ability were also better with donepezil but only by one point on a 60-point scale and this doesn't seem worth £1,000 [$2,000] per year."

And he could be thinking of the Rosofsky Law of Inverse Proportionality when he concludes: "Sadly, there are a lot of people with dementia and far too little money available to look after them. Doctors and health-care funders need to question whether it would be better to invest in more doctors and nurses and better social support rather than spending huge sums of money prescribing these expensive drugs. We need to develop more effective drugs than cholinesterase inhibitors. But, we shouldn't just focus on drugs—we also need to find more effective ways of supporting people with Alzheimer's disease and their carers."

The usual suspects had the usual reactions to this study—one that they didn't fund.

Pfizer said the sample was too small and the results inconsistent with previous results.

The Alzheimer's Association—drug companies pay for 5 percent of its budget—said the report "should not dictate individual treatment decisions," that families and doctors "working together" are in the best position to evaluate the effects of Aricept.

I'm sorry, but desperate anecdotal decisions are no substitute for double-blind science. They are no more compelling a testimonial for therapeutic effectiveness than would be a tale of a fifty-pound weight loss on a Wonder Bread diet.

Is this a corrupt system? Should we spend billions on dubious drugs rather than on people to hold the hands of the Alzheimer's afflicted?

I'm no neurobiological researcher, but I'm sure that any Alzheimer's cure will not include Aricept or Namenda. These drugs put cut flowers in water—prolonging the agony.

One morning I was drinking coffee, reading the paper, when on the front page I see: "Data About Zetia Risks Was Not Fully Revealed." Zetia is a cholesterol-fighting drug whose use I shared with millions. I saw the ads for this drug along with those for Viagra when I watched manly events like football. But its manufacturers, Merck and Schering-Plough, deep-sixed reports of liver damage. A Schering executive declared they didn't hide the data because it was unfavorable, but because they were "not scientifically important." I suspect Big Pharma makes calculations similar to Detroit: safer cars will be more expensive than paying off injury and death claims on unsafe cars.

In 2005, in the UK, the House of Commons Health Committee studied the web weaved by Big Pharma and concluded: "What has been described as the 'medicalisation' of society—the belief that every problem requires medical treatment—may also be attributed in part to the activities of the pharmaceutical industry. While the pharmaceutical industry cannot be blamed for creating unhealthy reliance on, and overuse of, medicines, it has certainly exacerbated it. There has been a trend towards categorizing more and more individuals as 'abnormal' or in need of drug treatment."

Overall, despite the occasional headline of a wrong foot amputation and the like, medicine gets great press. There are many fewer doctor jokes than lawyer jokes, and they tend to make fun of the godlike status of M.D.'s unlike the mocking of the sharklike status of lawyers. We tend to judge medicine by its heroic successes, of which there have been more than a few.

Diseases come and go, rise and fall, almost as if they were fashions like hemlines. When I was starting out in the 1970s, hyperactivity—now called attention deficit disorder—was hot. I had a stream of parents coming into my consultation room asking if they should put their obstreperous children on Ritalin or take them off Ritalin. When I was at all-female Mount Holyoke College, anorexia and bulimia were the rage. Later, depression became big. Autism is the disease du jour. It's in the moment. Along with a hot disease comes a social movement—or, at least an interest group. Celebrities who believe that the vaccine additive thermerosol causes autism are knocking on the doors of Congress demanding an end to its use—even as a British ban on thermerosol saw no subsequent decline in autism rates. Doesn't matter: it's my cause, and I'll cry if I want to.

I doubt these fads are the result of actual epidemiological

changes. Neither society nor human biology could have changed enough in the past few decades to account for an increase in autism. There are other, simpler explanations. Better diagnostic procedures and a greater awareness—due to publicity—bring forward parents wondering if their children are autistic. Look for something, and you will find what you're looking for. Follow the money. The federal government poured millions into the Individuals with Disabilities Education Act, and the increase in attention deficit disorders increased fivefold. New drugs appear to make more people sick. A more effective antidepressant one day, and the next you get millions of people—after watching ads on TV—saying, "Maybe that's what's wrong with me." Most medications, including antidepressants, are dispensed by primary care physicians, not by psychiatric experts. For many people, there's still a stigma in going to a psychiatric. It must mean they're crazy. It's easier to tell your family doctor you're feeling blue and walk out with a pill. No stigma attaches to your neighbor seeing you walking out of Dr. Welby's office.

Things do change. For most of my life there was no AIDS. Then it destroyed much of a generation—like World War I and the ensuing influenza epidemic. Deadly new diseases are typically infectious—not ineffable like depression or autism. Over time, some infections can be vanquished.

Karl Menninger made a starling observation when I heard him speak at the University of Chicago: "When I was a young medical student, most of the psychiatric patients I saw had late-stage syphilis." Menninger, born 1893, graduated from Harvard Medical School in 1917. This was ten years before Arthur Fleming discovered penicillin and a quarter of a century before the new antibiotic became a surefire cure for syphilis. Menninger's statement about syphilitic insanity—actually a type of dementia—clued me in that the world does change. A century ago unsafe sex could make you insane. A century later, millions of people secure in the knowledge that penicillin would cure syphilis blindly went to their deaths from AIDS. Dementia, too, has returned, but in a new package.

Until the twentieth century, human life expectancy averaged between twenty and thirty years, inching up to close to forty only for the more affluent in more developed countries. This is life expectancy calculated from infancy. Large numbers dropped like flies in childbirth, infancy, and childhood. Even so, in medieval times, if you reached twenty-five you could expect to live only to fifty. Women outliving men is a recent phenomenon. Many did not survive giving birth. Only recently did advances in public health, infection, and vaccination give rise to a quantum leap in longevity.

The flip side of increased life expectancy is that millions live long enough to develop conditions that were rare in previous eras. Before effective contraception, most women who were not nuns went through adulthood until death mostly pregnant. Today, a large majority of women go through their lives menstruating monthly. Menopause was rare, since most women were dead before its onset. Dementia has been around since ancient times, but it didn't become a public health problem until life expectancy caught up with old age.

A couple of months after my father moved to New Haven, at the age of eighty-six, he still knows he's he and I'm me, but he's already shaky on the past. I'm drinking supermarket orange juice at his kitchen table.

"This is not like the fresh-squeezed you got in Florida, Dad."

"Florida?"

"Don't you remember down in Florida?"

"I lived in Florida?"

"Yes. Century Village. West Palm Beach."

"I don't remember. There's something wrong with me. Something missing."

Sixty-three years before my father's birth, a girl called Auguste Deter was born in a small German village. In her forties, a typical hausfrau with one daughter, she began to demonstrate strange symptoms—memory loss, delusions, hallucinations, aphasia, catatonia, and rage. In 1901, at the Frankfurt Hospital for the Mentally Ill and Epileptics, a Dr. Alois Alzheimer examined her. Four years later, she died, and Alzheimer did a brain autopsy. He discovered abnormalities that remain the hallmarks of the disease that bears his name—buildups of protein inside and outside the nerve cells. These physical anomalies showed that dementia is not just an effect of aging—not all old people develop dementia and many younger people do.

Alzheimer's notes of his conversations with Auguste (translated by Konrad Maurer in a 1997 *Lancet* article), despite the passage of time, could seamlessly take their place alongside the notes of my own patient conversations.

On November 26, 1901, he wrote, "She sits on the bed with a helpless expression. What is your name? Auguste. Last name? Auguste. What is your husband's name? Auguste, I think. Your husband? Ah, my husband. She looks as if she didn't understand the question. Are you married? To Auguste. Mrs. D? Yes, yes, Auguste D. How long have you been here? She seems to be trying to remember. Three weeks. What is this? I show her a pencil. A pen. A purse and key, diary, cigar are identified correctly. At lunch she eats cauliflower and pork. Asked what she is eating she answers spinach. When she was chewing meat and asked what she was doing, she answered potatoes and then horseradish. When objects are shown to her, she does not remember after a short time which objects have been shown."

And on November 29 he wrote: "When she has to write Mrs. Auguste D, she writes Mrs. and we must repeat the other words because she forgets them. The patient is not able to progress in writing and repeats, I have lost myself."

My father: "Something is missing."

Although our understanding of Alzheimer's has increased a bit since Auguste's brain autopsy, we are as hopeless as ever in treating it. Palliative comfort and care is about the best we can offer—about the same as the clueless physicians in the face of the black death in the fourteenth century.

There are many kinds of dementia. Parkinson's and AIDS are just two of the diseases that yield dementia in their later stages. My father probably had vascular dementia, microstrokes starving his brain of oxygen. It's not easy to distinguish among the many types of dementia. There are no blood tests. No diagnostic brain scans. I can give you a psychological test and tell your family you have dementia but not tell them what kind. It's mostly guesswork until you die and someone cuts your skull open and examines your posthumous brain.

Alzheimer's is believed to account for 50 to 70 percent of all dementias. Vascular dementia and a type called Lewy body syndrome—associated with Parkinson's—account for around 15 percent each. The remaining dementias are rarer. But whatever kind you have, even if I could definitively diagnose the dementia of a living person, it wouldn't make much difference in treatment—there being little we can do except provide comfort for the afflicted and their families.

"Mrs. Ciccarelli, how's your memory?"

"It's great. I can remember back to kindergarten."

This is typical. Early memories are well-trodden paths through the forest of the brain. It's remembering what you had for breakfast that can be dicey. It's a less-trodden path. Simple forgetting is not the problem—like when you can't remember where you put your keys. When you forget you forgot your keys, you have a problem. I reassure the nondemented by saying it's good you remember breakfast, even if you forget what you ate.

People who know who they are, what's the date, and where they are, we call oriented times three—person, time, and place. For people slipping into dementia, time orientation is usually the first to go. Next to go is being able to identify the location.

"Mrs. Ciccarelli, what's the date?"

"You would have to ask me that, but I stopped paying attention. I can tell you Mrs. Green was my first-grade teacher."

"Mrs. Ciccarelli, what town are we in?"

"Harrisburg."

We're sitting in a small town in Connecticut.

Mrs. Ciccarelli lived most of her life in Harrisburg, until she had a slip and a fall and her daughter insisted she take up residence in a nursing home near her in Connecticut.

Mrs. Emma Ciccarelli still knows she is Mrs. Emma Ciccarelli, that she has two daughters, one of whom she doesn't talk to anymore, and that there's a bunch of grandchildren, and a couple of great-grandchildren. It's January, and after saying hello, I chitchat about what nice weather we're having for winter. She agrees, and

155

NASTY, BRUTISH, AND LONG

tells me she went for Christmas dinner to the home of the daughter with whom she is speaking. Yet when I ask her the date, a few minutes later, she has no idea.

"Is it August?"

Two or three years from this encounter, she might forget she has any daughters, her own name, and, eventually—if she lives long enough—she might look at food and not know it's for eating.

As one of my professors said about Hegel, I can say about the inevitable losses of dementia, "We'll peel away the layers of the onion until there is nothing left but the smell."

If we were Nazis, we would kill all the people with dementia. Before they came for the Jews, the Germans killed the demented. Soon after their rise to power in 1933, they began sterilizing what Hitler called "diseased elements" of society. The leader of the fatherland had a compulsive attitude about health, and viewed society through a medicalized disease model. People with congenital feeble-mindedness, schizophrenia, manic depression, hereditary epilepsy, Huntington's chorea, hereditary blindness, hereditary deafness, and serious physical deformities were sterilized so as to cleanse future generations of their taint. This was not purely a Nazi attitude. Eugenics—the view that we should encourage the fit to reproduce and the unfit not to—was part of the common culture. None other than Alexander Graham Bell—in his role as teacher of the deaf—advocated their sterilization. A supposedly progressive president, Woodrow Wilson—who brought his southern racial attitudes to the White House—supported the movement, as did Sir Francis Galton, Margaret Sanger, H. G. Wells, and George Bernard

Shaw. Not all these eugenicists advocated sterilization. Instead, many encouraged smart people like you and me to reproduce more. But the hardcore managed to sterilize 65,000 retarded, mentally ill, and physically deformed citizens in the United States—as well as passing marriage laws preventing people with certain conditions, like epilepsy, from marrying. The Germans did surpass us, sterilizing 400,000 before they started World War II in 1939.

After the war began, they kicked it up more than a few notches with Action T4. A very organized and record-driven people, they required the unanimous vote of three doctors to lethally inject or starve to death more than 100,000 children and adults—people who previously had been only sterilized. The list for euthanasia included old people with dementia—the type of people I work with every day. Sterilizing people who couldn't reproduce anyway had nothing to do with eugenics, but it did save money. The Nazi propaganda machine treated the "diseased elements" much the way some of us think about illegal aliens, as a drain on the healthy elements of society. One poster put at 60,000 deutsche marks the amount of treasure that the typical defective stole from society.

This program ended in 1941. Good Germans, who had few problems with killing my relatives, were not happy about killing their own "defective" but loved relatives. The cessation of Action T4 was one of the few successful opposition movements under the Nazis.

In our more humane society, we're distressed that dementia costs the functional equivalent of 60,000 deutsche marks. But instead of traveling down euthanasia's cheap road, we spend our treasure on Big Pharma's chemical restraints. We calculate it is cheaper than going drug free and spending the savings on staffing and supportive environments. We're too moral to kill them off, but too cheap to give them a collective group hug. Who wants higher taxes?

It's not only the marginally effective antidementia drugs that soak up the money. We spend billions more on chemical restraints. Most of the dementia patients I know take powerful antipsychotic medications. The doctor who prescribed Depakote for my father subtly implied it would be hard to keep him in the institution if they didn't medicate him. I should have called his bluff—Dad out on the sidewalk in his wheelchair—surrounded by his luggage. Demented confusion aside, the homes get antsy about rage, hallucinations, and delusions. I met a woman last week who insisted there were bugs crawling all over her bed—and this in a very hygienic facility—and another who calmly let on we were in a factory and she had to get back to the assembly line because break was over. But she added, "It's a very nice factory. I like working here."

The antipsychotic meds currently in vogue—Zyprexa, Seroquel, Risperdal, Abilify—were designed and approved for the treatment of schizophrenia. I love how they brand these drugs—giving the Anglophile nursing home names a run for their money. Seroquel with its "Ser" for serene and "quel" for reducing to submission. Abilify, which is some kind of nonsensical neologism—making up nonsense words is a hallmark of schizophrenia—is supposed to conjure up some profound yet ineffable action on the mind.

It wasn't long after their development that psychiatrists wondered whether drugs for reducing the hallucinations and delusions of schizophrenia would also do the same for the hallucinations and delusions of dementia. This "off label" use ran up against the finding that elderly patients taking antipsychotics are more than twice as likely to suffer death from respiratory or cardiac failure. The

FDA issued this warning: "None [of the antipsychotics] is approved for the treatment of behavioral disorders in patients with dementia. Because of these findings, the Agency will ask the manufacturers of these drugs to include a Boxed Warning in their labeling describing this risk and noting that these drugs are not approved for this indication." This means more opportunity for lawyers, since they didn't ban the drugs, only certified them as dangerous. These risks, medical and legal, haven't stopped their wide use among the institutionalized elderly: "The bottom line is that with this patient group there are times when these drugs have to be used, and there are currently no alternatives," psychiatrist Roger Bullock told *Neuropsychiatry Reviews.*

The bottom line for the legal profession is my vision of a lawyer waving the FDA warning in front of a defendant doctor, "You knew about this, didn't you, doctor, before you gave Seroquel to that poor dear dead old lady?"

And it's not only the antipsychotics and the antidementia drugs that they give to the dear old ladies. There are the antidepressants, the tranquilizers, the sleeping pills, and the antianxiety drugs. It's not uncommon for a nursing home resident to be on all of these, plus whatever drugs they take for their variety of physical ailments. I'm servicing a drugged-out, hyped-up population. Filling out my forms, I often run out of the space provided for the list of drugs. There's a technical term for this: "polypharmacy." Most of the people I see qualify. It's no wonder that someone taking half a dozen pills or more several times a day will need the services of a careful nurse to keep up with the pill burden. And I can't help but wondering whether a big hug or, failing that, a slug of whiskey might do just as well.

Some people call the psychiatrist's bluff.

I'm at Bothwell Bridge Assisted Living Center. They're asking me to see Moses Rabinowitz. In the chart, a note: "No psych meds."

"Mr. Rabinowitz sits in his room all day," the nurse tells me.

"What's he in for?" I ask—inadvertently with the prison slang.

"He's eighty-eight and his family thought he shouldn't be on his own."

"So what's the problem?"

"He just sits in his room all day. Like I told you."

She sounds exasperated.

"What's this about no psych meds?"

"Well, the family doesn't want to drug him out. But we convinced them to allow you to talk to him."

Occasionally this happens—this drug resistance. Maybe there was a previous bad experience with psychotropic drugs. Maybe they're opposed on principle. You don't have to be a Scientologist to be against psych drugs. I know people who don't vaccinate their kids. The Rabinowitzes probably think it's harmless enough to have their dad talk to me.

I open up the Rabinowitz chart. Flip through the pages. First, of course, I check that he has Medicare. If he has managed care, it's a hassle. I can't see him right away, and it could be weeks before we get approval. Then I turn to the social history. Widower for twelve years. Lived in his house for more than fifty years. A raised ranch. Better that he had a pure ranch, absent even those few steps in and out of the living room. He's from Brooklyn—a *landsman*. Even went to my college, where he studied accounting. Quite an accomplishment for a Depression boy.

My father managed to finish three years of college at St. John's University, a Catholic school no less. He was studying accounting too. He liked to tell me how he made the dean's list and the dean called him a fine student. Came over to shake his hand. Then poverty got the better of his plans, a few years before World War II further intervened. I don't know why he didn't finish his degree after the war on the GI Bill. So close—only a year or two to go. Perhaps it was my mother's pressure. "Get a job!" Or the pressure of supporting newborn me. One of those mysteries I'll never solve. If he had finished, my dad could have been like Mr. Rabinowitz, an accountant, a comptroller of a leading cardboard box company, living in suburbia, the raised ranch, a new car—like clockwork—every three years. And I could have had a more happy childhood, become an accountant too, lacking imagination—no dreams of writing.

I interrupt these reveries and flip the pages to the medical section. Not only does Rabinowitz have a clean bill of health—save for the hearing aids and lower back pain. Not only is he not taking any psych meds, he's taking no meds at all. I'm surprised. Instead of flipping casually through the medical pages, I turn them slowly and read them carefully one by one. I do this several times. Front to back. Back to front. We have a winner. It's rare but it happens—the med sheet not looking like a formulary.

I walk into Mr. Rabinowitz's room.

"Who are you?"

"My name is Ira, and I'm a psychologist. I'd just like to talk with you a bit."

"Who sent you?"

"Your doctor, Dr. Mukterjee."

"I've never met him."

"And your daughter thought it might not be a bad idea."

"All right. Sit down. If I don't talk to you, she'll give me hell."

We chat about Brooklyn, although neither of us has lived there for large chunks of a century. I find he had a class with the philosopher Morris Raphael Cohen at City College. Long gone, yet legendary by the time I was there majoring in philosophy.

We are both enjoying ourselves. The shared ethnicity. The shared cultural background. I tell him I majored in philosophy.

"I would have done that, but I had to make a living to justify the family sacrifice of my being there."

"So, Mr. Rabinowitz, in your own words, what brings you here?"

"It's my son-in-law. He's retiring and they're moving to Florida. I'm one hundred percent healthy, but he—only sixty-three—is diabetic, already had a heart attack. My daughter would worry about me all alone in the house. So here I am.

"I think about moving down there too, near them. But what would I do in Florida? Hate the place. But my daughter says, once she gets settled, maybe she'll find a place for me. We'll see."

"So why did you come here?"

"My house is in the middle of nowhere. I don't drive. And my chauffeur is going to Florida. I can't get too mad. After all, I abandoned my own mother to New York City years ago, when I moved to Connecticut."

Just like me.

Unlike me is Emily Jones—a rural Connecticut farm girl. Now, she is seventy-three, her four children are scattered to the wind—except for the one who is buried nearby, twenty-odd years after he succumbed to a drug overdose—and her husband is at another nursing home with dementia. Her childhood farm is long gone to a housing development, part of humanity's inexorable destruction of the natural world. Today, as always, Mrs. Jones is restless with pain. Her life—whether in bed or wheelchair—is a constant search for a position in which she can find a minimum amount of pain for a maximum amount of time. Her main affliction is idiopathic neuropathy. To this, we can add high cholesterol, hypertension, gastroesophageal reflux disease, macular degeneration, gout, and depression. It's the pain, though, that drives and suffuses her existence.

"How are you today?"

"I just can't get comfortable."

This day, I find her in bed. She's a constant torment of movement. She can sigh like a Jew. I even hear an "Oy!" from this daughter of the soil.

Her meds reflect her afflictions: Lipitor, Lasix, Zestril, Protonix, Lucentis, Ambien, Ativan, and Lexapro. She's a gold mine for Big Pharma. From Little Pharma—over-the-counter meds—she's popping nonsteroidal anti-inflammatory medications—Aleve, Motrin—several times a day.

"Nothing is helping!" she implores. "I'm hot. I'm cold. I'm tingling all over. Oh, the pain!"

In their progress notes, the nurses make noises about "drug-seeking behavior," but who am I to judge? I can witness but can't feel her pain.

Neuropathy is a disease of the peripheral nervous system, the network running throughout our bodies that sends messages to and from the brain. In Mrs. Jones's case it's idiopathic, meaning they don't know what's behind it. Idiopathic means peculiar to the individual. As the dictionary says, "from an obscure or unknown cause." As the bumper sticker says, "Shit happens."

For Mrs. Jones, it means she can't get no satisfaction, no matter how much she tries. It also means she embodies a medical paradox. When I hear "drug-seeking behavior," it usually means someone looking to kill the pain. Docs don't have a problem loading up people with drugs—antidepressants, tranquilizers, diuretics, statins, acetylcholinesterase inhibitors—but when you get to the point of controlled substances they run scared. Morphine and other opiates—all originally derived from the poppy—are wonders against pain. During the American Civil War—that meat grinder of attrition—hundreds of thousands of wounded soldiers found relief in morphine; no more just biting the bullet. In the nineteenth century, laudanum—liquid opium—sold like aspirin. Brands included Mrs. Winslow's Wonder Drops, guaranteed to soothe your cranky baby. The drug wars begun in the twentieth century failed against alcohol, but had successes in the fight against morphine. The average primary care physician, who wouldn't think twice about prescribing powerful psychotropic drugs like antidepressants, is quite reluctant to prescribe morphine. They're afraid the authorities will go after them if they chalk up too many narcotic prescriptions. I can attest to morphine's effectiveness. Following my surgery, I bravely told people I had no pain. That is, until they stopped the morphine, and then, "Ouch!"

For the most part, the use of narcotics is confined to a short period after surgery and the short period before death. If your pain is long-term, you get to suffer long-term.

Pain management with narcotics has largely been relegated to pain management specialists—mostly anesthesiologists. There is kind of a gentleman's agreement. Let specialists, and only specialists, prescribe the controlled substances and no one will get prosecuted.

Narcotics aside, there's research that indicates a good hit or two of marijuana may be even more effective against neuropathic pain. But that has a whole other set of problems. No nursing home—

worried about a long list of governmental regulations—is going to take the risk of providing a bong or brownies for Mrs. Jones. In nursing home culture, a scheduled sexual orgy is more likely than passing a joint around a circle of wheelchairs. There is a pharmaceutical form of marijuana, Marinol, but it's very expensive and rarely prescribed.

It's the fear of addiction that drives the fear of narcotics. It's not that simple. True, you will likely develop a physical dependence when you take narcotics, but if you are not prone to addiction, a tapering down of the drug will alleviate the discomfort of withdrawal and you won't have the craving to go back to it. You will also develop tolerance, which means that a given dosage will not alleviate your pain. To a pain management specialist, this means increase the dosage until it's effective, not stop it. And a high dosage of narcotics for Emily Jones's pain is typically many times less than the amount an addict takes for his deeper kind of psychic pain.

If there is a scandal here, it's the fact that millions of pain sufferers get no relief. The American College of Physicians estimated that half of all cancer patients, for example, feel they are receiving inadequate pain treatment.

I suggest a pain management referral for Emily Jones, but it never seems to happen. Specialists don't make house or nursing home calls. So, instead, I continue to hear her sighs along with the sighs of the staff. "We just gave you a Motrin an hour ago, Emily."

Even if you get pain meds, they might cut you off at the knees.

I'm back at Hasting Manor for my weekly session with Benjamin Cardozo Lombardi—his mother thought the noted jurist was Italian. He sits in his wheelchair, and his left foot is gone. His right foot is still with us, but missing its toes. He has type 2 diabetes, which is associated with, but not necessarily caused by, old age. There are big numbers here. An estimated 20 percent of people over age sixty-five have type 2, non-insulin-dependent diabetes. We don't understand why the pancreas starts shutting down after a lifetime of service for so many people. Mr. Lombardi had all the warning signs—obesity, high blood pressure, high cholesterol. His mother had diabetes too. But this constellation of warning signs does not constitute a cause. Like Mrs. Jones, he also has neuropathy, diabetic neuropathy. Thirty percent of those with type 2 diabetes develop neuropathy. Poor circulation—characteristic of diabetes—damaged the nerves in Mr. Lombardi's legs. You might feel nothing. You could walk around for a day with a nail through your foot and not feel a thing. Lombardi developed the characteristic ulcers, which became infected, and they started lopping off the appendages.

"I feel like a salami. A slice here and a slice there." Reminds me of Drake McHugh (Ronald Reagan) in *Kings Row*: "Where's the rest of me?"

The nursing home is a realm of withering and rotting, I have to say.

This is not the terrain of the institutionalized psychotic youth I traveled through in my early career. Those teenagers might have been hallucinating, rocking, screaming, but their bizarre behavior retained the bloom of youth. That crazy girl was a beautiful and young crazy girl. Now it's amputation, sunken runny eyes, sores, stooped bodies, wrinkly, parched leathery skin, and blood blisters. It brings to mind the cut flowers out of water (or in water), or the abandoned peach one of my kids left behind in the backseat of my car. The way of all flesh—animal and vegetable.

My mother called me one evening after a visit to her cardiologist. "Ira, I ask him why I feel so bad and he tells me I'm old. What should I expect?" he asks. "Ira, I expect an explanation."

Add aging to the long list of medical mysteries. It's one of those puzzles like Why do we need to sleep? or Why can't you tickle yourself? The most satisfying explanation I've heard for sleep is evolutionary. Evolving humans slept to remove themselves from harm's way. By crawling into a cave or climbing a tree and dozing off, they became less likely targets for nighttime predators against whom they had little defense.

There is an evolutionary aspect to aging and its eventual end— death. If we didn't die, there would be no room for new generations. We'd be old-growth forests where the only living trees are old trees casting shadows on young saplings struggling for the light.

Isaac Asimov imagined a society where people lived indefinitely. Each of them lives in paranoid isolation—like Howard Hughes or J. D. Salinger—communicating only via videophones. Human contact brings the ills that flesh is heir to. Their only companions are robots. These people don't reproduce. Their personal yet reclusive longevity threatens the survival of the species.

But why we in the world of non–science fiction reality age rather than simply keel over and die in the bloom of youth remains an unknown. There is the theory that our cells and their DNA are copy machines—indefinitely making copies of themselves. Take a photo of your face and copy it, then copy the copy, and so on. After a million times, your face would take on a new aspect. All those little errors adding up. Your photo would age like the portrait of Dorian Gray.

There are other theories. That there is some kind of biological clock for aging. That waste products build up in our cells. That we are machines that simply wear out over time. Pick one. Your guess is as good as mine or any expert researcher's. Aging is a young science.

Mens sana in corpore sano. A sound mind in a sound body.

If you have both, you will not be in a nursing home. If you don't have one or the other, you probably will be.

I often wonder, and sometimes even ask a patient who can appreciate the question: would you prefer to have dementia but be physically healthy, or would you like all your marbles in an ailing body? Either is a bad bargain. Do you want full awareness of your frailty, pain, and suffering? Or would you want to be addled but fit to ambulate purposelessly down the halls of the nursing home? Complainer that I am, I would still choose the sound mind in the unsound body—although it depends on how unsound.

My dog appears perfectly happy lying on the couch near me by the fire in January, but does he know—is he conscious—that he is happy? The pleasantly confused type of dementia lacks human awareness. As the parts of the brain that underlie our self-consciousness are destroyed, we are left with animal awareness without the animal's skills for survival. A human with serious dementia has the real-world survival skills of a Pekingese dog, which were bred by the Chinese to sit on laps, look like miniature lions, and not much else.

Although our understanding of aging is limited, we can easily enumerate its afflictions: chronic obstructive pulmonary disorder, diabetes, macular degeneration, glaucoma, heart disease, gastro-esophageal reflux disease, strokes, gout, arthritis, Parkinson's, cancer, and osteoporosis. Common to these conditions is the lack of any real cure. These are not infections, for which antibiotics can bring a reversal. For the most part, these are chronic conditions that we can manage but not eliminate. It is ironic that so many of the nursing homes label themselves health care centers, when disease care centers would be far more accurate—but admittedly bad for marketing.

These diseases are common among the old, but we can't say that old age is either a necessary or a sufficient cause of them. People much younger than me have cancer, Parkinson's, and even osteoporosis. And people older than me have a clean bill of health. I have no access to the medical records of Walter Cronkite, but if he has any of these illnesses, they don't seem to be impeding his sailing his sixty-four-foot yacht, *Wyntje*. I have to remind myself again and again that the sick people I see confined in the institution are a slice of life, not the slice shared by all their peers.

In the nursing home, I walk each day through the terrain of medical care. There are oxygen tanks, IV machines, various kinds of wheelchairs, various kinds of beds, and the cyclical progression of the med pass nurse working her way up and down the halls.

The nursing home looks like a hospital, but it is also the workshop of entropy. Time's arrow leading us to disorder and chaos. All of us worker bees moving on the assembly line from room to room. Each of us turning a screw, emplacing a widget, removing a blemish—fingers in the dike against disease.

"Mr. Harrelson, I see you have oxygen. How long has that been?"

"Since I came here, a couple of weeks ago."

"Did you smoke?"

"I did, but I quit."

"It's always a good idea. When did you quit?"

"Oh, a couple of weeks ago. When I came here."

He's been there for a year. But he knows precisely that it's January 16, 2008, and that he was born in 1926.

"How old are you, sir."

"Somewhere in my fifties."

"Who is the current president?"

"Reagan."

"And who was the president before him?"

"Carter."

It does fit together in a kind of coherence. He says he's fiftyish and those were the presidents when he actually was fifty.

"I'm very sorry to hear about your wife."

She died last week.

"It was sad," said with surprising dispassion.

"I'll be back to talk to you from time to time."

"That would be nice."

I mark down "rule out denial." It's my feeble attempt at understanding his apparent lack of grief—as I turn my own little screw in the production line.

The nurses say Mrs. Solomon is apathetic. I find her lying in bed, eyes closed, mouth wide open. We chat about the weather. It's January. She thinks it's June. It gives you some idea of how her mind works when the trees are bare, snow is falling, and she thinks it's June—even as she gazes out the window.

"Are you going to therapy?"

"I did go, but they said I graduated."

When I came into her room I turned down the TV. When I'm leaving, I ask her if she wants the TV back on.

"No, I'm just going to nap now."

Even though she thinks it's June when it's January, she well knows that graduating physical therapy means they expect no further progress. She probably knows that the rehab stay her daughter promised will be lifelong.

Of course, not everyone in the home has a terminal sentence. The usual scenario is hospitalization followed by the nursing home for rehabilitation. You break your hip. You have pneumonia. You go to the nursing home but have a shot at home sweet home. When they use the word "therapy" in the nursing home, they're not thinking about a consultation with Dr. Rosofsky.

It's easy to think of physical therapy as something real. I peer in at the typical setup and I see residents lifting free weights, climbing up and down a small flight of stairs, pulling at colorful muscle-strengthening elastic bands, walking down the hall with a staff person—often in the uniform of khaki pants and color polo shirt complete with logo, like that of a cell phone salesman—holding them up, getting in and out of chairs, transferring from a bed to a chair, getting their arms manipulated up and down. Going to therapy in the morning is often a convenient reason to want to nap all afternoon. "They worked me out this morning and now I'm bushed."

Both short-term and long-term patients get physical therapy. If you're going home—and for a particular illness or accident all Medicare payments stop after one hundred days—we want to help you get home before the payments stop. And if you are never going home, we want you to use your walker or being able to go the bathroom by yourself as much as possible.

All this activity going on—the grunting, the sighing, the encouraging "Go for it," which is what I heard when they encouraged terrified, foolish me to rappel backward off a four-hundred-foot-high

NASTY, BRUTISH, AND LONG

cliff at Outward Bound—and it's easy to imagine that it's all for the good, that something real is happening.

It calls to mind the funeral director in Cathy Pelletier's *Once upon a Time on the Banks* who frets that fitness programs in nursing homes are slowing down his business.

Physical therapy is a booming multibillion-dollar industry. According to the Bureau of Labor Statistics (BLS), in 2006 there were 173,000 physical therapists. About a third work in nursing homes, along with tens of thousands of unlicensed aides requiring no college degree. The demand will only increase. "The increasing elderly population will drive growth in the demand for physical therapy services. The elderly population is particularly vulnerable to chronic and debilitating conditions that require therapeutic services. Also, the baby-boom generation is entering the prime age for heart attacks and strokes, increasing the demand for cardiac and physical rehabilitation," reports the BLS. Want your son or daughter to train for a job with security that requires only a bachelor's degree and will net them close to a six-figure salary along with professional respect? Physical therapy could be the ticket.

But as long ago as 1969, Eugene Michel, the president of the American Physical Therapy Association, gave a speech to his membership calling upon physical therapists to stop relying on personal intuition, training, suggestions of mentors and colleagues, and to start relying on scientific research to shape their clinical practice. After this, evidence-based practice became a preoccupation of physical therapy. There were several barriers to this science-minded approach. First and foremost was the absence of much research supporting one procedure over another. In the decades since Michel's address, there has been a fair amount of research—facilitated by the development of doctoral level physical therapy programs. However, evidence-based practice, in practice, remains a problem.

One review of 179 journal articles found that only 11 percent "met the criteria of high-quality evidence suitable for direct application to patient care."

When I reviewed some of the supposedly quality physical therapy research I found it to be suggestively similar to the Aricept and Namenda research. For example, "Effects of Extended Outpatient Rehabilitation After Hip Fracture," published in the *Journal of the American Medical Association*, looked at a very common cause of injury to the elderly and compared a supervised physical therapy program—involving progressive resistance training—to a low-impact home exercise program. The researchers note that "only a small number of controlled studies have been conducted of rehabilitation interventions after hip fracture"—indicating a lack of evidence to buttress evidence-based physical therapy practice. The study found statistically significant differences between the two groups—home exercise and physical therapy—but the differences were quite small. In other words, physical activity is good, and physical therapy might be a tad better.

I wonder whether the role of the physical therapist is to provide a safe environment for exercise, assuring compliance, but not much more. I also wonder whether post-fracture, my dad would have improved—even after graduating from physical therapy—if only the aides had actually taken him on supervised walks.

Evidence for evidence-based practice aside, reviews of how physical therapists make treatment decisions appear not to have changed greatly since Michel gave his speech in 1969. According to a 2005 literature review by Joe Schreiber and Perri Stern: "Despite numerous calls for a shift toward the use of research and scientific evidence to guide practice, most physical therapists continued to base practice decisions largely on anecdotal evidence, and utilized treatment techniques with little scientific support. Studies published in

1997 and 1999 indicated that physical therapists tended to rely more heavily on initial education and training when selecting treatment techniques. In fact, less than five percent of survey respondents indicated that they regularly used scientific evidence to guide practice. Personal experience and 'expert' opinion guided clinical decision making throughout the 1990s."

I don't mean to pick on physical therapists. I have no doubt that other clinicians—me included—are guilty of the sins of relying on initial education, anecdotal evidence, and using treatment techniques with little scientific support.

Consider Freud, for example. Freud was a great writer, a bold, imaginative, revolutionary thinker, but face it, his research method, the case study, is purely anecdotal. For decades, hardheaded thinkers gained tenure by, essentially, making fun of the psychoanalytic case study method and its lack of testable hypotheses. Psychoanalysts would often defend themselves—somewhat circularly—by accusing their detractors of having psychological problems. And they would argue you have to be part of the process to understand its effectiveness. Freud thought big thoughts, but today researchers look at small, incremental factors—not whether therapy cures childhood trauma, but whether talking to someone will make patients report they are feeling better.

In the end, when I look at the nursing home I am reduced to the provisional conclusion that lots of people spending lots of time with the residents—be they psychologists, nurses, physical therapists, doctors, aides, custodial staff, recreational therapists, and shrinks like me—can only be a good thing. The obverse of the Rosofsky Law of Inverse Proportionality.

THE FINAL CHAPTER

Dying and Death

’m sitting around the house minding my own business. The phone rings. It’s the physician assistant at Dad’s nursing home.

“Your father is very sick. He’s going to die, and there’s nothing you can do about it.”

Talk about bedside manner. I’m wondering why she said there’s nothing I can do about it when she’s the one on the job, but what I say is, “What do you mean?”

“I mean he’s very sick and going to die.”

She’s telling me there’s nothing to do, but I do what I can. “I’ll be right over.”

At nursing homes, there’s silence about death. It’s the overlooked, uninvited thirteenth fairy who condemns you to eternity. But this is no fairy tale; there’s no good fairy to induce a coma instead of death, and no Prince Charming to revive you with a kiss.

Nobody “dies” in a nursing home. The euphemistic leitmotif for all things eldercare extends to the final chapter. Recently, I walked into a nursing home with a referral to see Joyce Bellanino. I can't find Bellanino.

"Where's the Bellanino chart?" I ask one of the nurses.

"Oh, she passed."

"Passed," "expired," "gone" are the usual euphemisms. We're too secular to say that Joyce Bellanino has gone to her reward, and we're not flip or hard-boiled enough to say she's kicked the bucket or having a dirt nap or the big sleep. We keep it pleasant and innocuous.

There is little memorialization. Some homes have a party for each month's birthday boys and girls, but I've never seen a memorial service for the passed and expired. The other day I saw a little obituary—a paid listing—for a woman I had met a couple of times. Someone had posted it on the bulletin board behind the nursing station. My act of remembrance was to read it. Mother of four. On the production line at Pratt & Whitney for twenty-five years. Predeceased by her husband. Wake tomorrow night. Burial Friday. And so she passes into history. I'm sure the obit will be gone the next time I show up. On the counter, her chart is being deconstructed, an empty binder sits next to its innards—a thick stack of paper on its way to its own burial in the records room. Next week, the binder will be reborn, filling up with paper for a new resident in my little world of aging, dying, and death.

On the chart's face sheet is one space for religion, and one for a funeral home. In New Haven, ethnicity traditionally dictates church attendance, not only Catholic, Protestant, and Jew, but finer distinctions such as St. Mary's for the Irish, St. Stanislaus for the Polish, and St. Anthony's for the Italians. These lifelong choices are reflected in the funeral home chart entries—Clancy's, Lupinski's, and Celentano's. Around the corner from where I live is a funeral home for Yankees. There are still Connecticut Yankees in Connecticut, but it shares its space with one of the Jewish undertakers. When the time comes, they could easily trundle me over on a gurney—no hearse required.

Listing the funeral home on the face sheet of the chart is convenient. The staff knows whom to call. After a death, I'll see a couple of sturdy young men in dark suits enter a room where the curtain is drawn around the bed, and leave it wheeling a cart with a cloth-covered corpse. They manage this with a minimum of fuss, often when the residents are at lunch or asleep. Never through the lobby. Always a side or back door. We don't want to upset the residents, unless you're the young man I met in a nursing home who was waiting for someone anonymous to die so he could claim the kidney. He had the misfortune that his less-than-anonymous roommate did die: "I had to spend the night with a dead body, right next to me! I've never been with a dead person before."

Among the dead people I've seen, few were in nursing homes, and those mostly behind curtains and under sheets. After catching a glimpse of my dead grandmother when I was five or six, I didn't see a dead person in person until I met my wife—not to say Linda was dead. I attended her family wakes and saw bodies all dressed up in a coffin with only one place to go. I saw the parade of condolers at the wakes, most genuflecting before the earthly remains. Then they would approach the reception line of mourners before saying, "He looks so good," or "He's not suffering anymore." We Jews go for the closed coffin. You die and you're already a memory. Most of us have to take it on faith that there is a body in there. When my mother died, I learned it wasn't just a matter of faith. There are the stories of undertakers who sell off body parts and whole bodies, and bury empty coffins or substitute kitty litter for cremated ashes. To insure there was no fraud in the case of my mother, the funeral director called my brother and me over to the hearse, lifted the lid, and we identified Mom. No fraud here. "Yes, that's her." Except that it wasn't. It was her body.

Or as a female patient of mine who had issues with men and relationships said: "One of these days I'd like to shoot one of my boyfriends. One minute a human, the next minute chemicals."

Mom died all of a sudden. There was none of this "Your father is going to die, and you can't do anything about it" business. I called her every day, in her mind a poor substitute for living with me, but the best I could do. One Monday, in a rush, I told her I was on my way out to see my kids in their school pageant.

"Have a good time," she said—not too bad a statement for what turned out to be her final words to me.

The next day, I received a call from my cousin.

"Your mother's in the hospital."

"Huh? Why? How is she doing?"

My cousin found out because her own mother—my aunt, my mother's ninety-three-year-old sister—was in the hospital too.

"One of the neighbors came by, and there was no answer, so they got the super to open the door, and she was passed out on the floor. I don't know how it's going now. I'll get back to you soon."

I call around the hospital, don't make much progress. I don't want to tie up my phone. It's 1997, before my cell phone or e-mail days. The phone rings. It's my cousin.

"I'm so sorry, Ira, Aunt Rebecca passed away."

My mother had been granted her wish. She and my Aunt Estelle were the two surviving children of her family. My mother once confided to Linda an abiding fear of being all alone, the last to die, without any of her three big sisters to dote on her. Now it would not be a problem.

The next day, my brother picks me up on his way from Boston and we drive to the apartment. In the TV room—once my room—there are the remains of her final day—a cup of tea gone cold, a cut-up apple gone brown, life receding. Out the window of this sixth-floor apartment there's a clear view over Brooklyn rooftops into Manhattan. It's 1998, and I admire yet again the Twin Towers of the World Trade Center. You could sit in the chair and see them peeping over the top of the TV before they came tumbling down.

Freud began his intellectual journey with the drive for pleasure—Eros—and its modulation by experience and society underlying all human behavior. But as he neared his own end, he reflected on the human capacity for self-destruction and concluded that the death drive—Thanatos—deserved an equal place. It was not an accident that he proposed this in 1920, when he was about my age, in *Beyond the Pleasure Principle*. World War I with its millions of willful deaths had recently concluded; traumatized veterans were entering his consultation room. It's commonplace to think the will to preserve life overrides all, but this is obviously not true. There's suicide; there's self-mutilation; there's a sexual fetish where near-suffocation intensifies orgasms; and there's war and genocide.

In his 1920 book, Freud wrote that the death drive works to "reestablish a state of things that was disturbed by the emergence of life"—death as quiescence. Freud grew up in a time shortly after the Second Law of Thermodynamics was postulated, in 1850—the idea, also known as entropy, that active physical systems, left undisturbed, will end in a state of quiescence. Turn the heat off under bubbling, boiling water and it becomes quiet and lukewarm.

Seen this way, the nursing home is the workshop of entropy and Thanatos. Left undisturbed, the lives I see would soon fall into their own private quiescence. We health care workers are a brake against this inevitability. At my still relatively young age, I have to come to grips with my own end. I do the math on life expectancy, and with each year it adds up to an increasingly smaller number. Yet I still find it hard to understand what so many of my elders tell me: "Enough already. I'm ready to go."

Fear of death is never a cause for referral to me, but we youngsters continue to project our will to live onto our elders' drive toward quiescence. When someone tells the nurse he is ready to go, she refers him to me for suicidal ideation. Since when did thinking—ideating—about death become suicidal fantasy? We reformulate the ideation by calling it depression—although who am I to call a ninety-year-old man in pain, in sickness, and in an institution depressed, rather than someone having an appropriate reaction to an unenviable situation?

Perhaps it is because he came from Hungary—historically, the country with the world's highest suicide rates—that Thomas Szasz, a psychiatrist who is paradoxically the leader of the antipsychiatry movement, considers suicide a fundamental human right. In the article "On the Future of Psychotherapy," published in the journal *The New Therapist*, Szasz writes: "I use the term 'psychotherapy' as the name of a freely contracted relationship between two competent and responsible adults, one paying the other for assisting him, by means of a dialogue, to live his life better." In this light, he sees "treatment" as coercive "harm that people seek to impose on others." The therapist should not "prescribe drugs, prevent suicide, or otherwise interfere with the patient's life." And he notes with dismay a legal situation in which the withholding of so-called "essential treatment" is unethical and illegal.

Many of Szasz's ideas about individual autonomy and the right to suicide have begun to creep into our common culture. He rejects the idea of state-sanctioned euthanasia—believing that suicide is a private act that should neither be sanctioned nor prohibited by the government—and the Netherlands has essentially followed the Szaszian decriminalization route. For years, physician-assisted suicide, to relieve intractable suffering, has been an element of Dutch medical practice. Since 2002, the country has immunized physicians from prosecution if they follow these guidelines: the patient is competent to make the request for assistance; the suffering is irreversible; and a physician peer reviews the request. This does not quite go the full-fledged route of Szasz, who sees suicide as a right irrespective of "suffering," but it allows physicians to enable the death wishes of patients in nursing homes (or outside nursing homes) who don't have the means or the physical ability to do themselves in.

In the United States, the rate of suicide throughout the life span remains quite low for women—less than ten per hundred thousand. For men, it rises significantly as they age—from less than ten per hundred thousand among adolescents, to between twenty and thirty throughout most adulthood, to a high of more than sixty per hundred thousand among elderly males. I'm not sure how to interpret these gender differences. I know that men with their violent means tend to be more successful at killing themselves than women—a gun to the head is more likely to succeed than a bottle of pills—so the death wish may be the same. Putting aside the gender differences, suicide rates among people sixty-five and older are the highest for any age group. Composing only 12 percent of the population, the elderly overachievers account for 16 percent of suicide deaths.

Inside the nursing home, the desire to put an end to one's life may be as high—if not higher—than on the outside. But the actual rates are quite low, if not immeasurable. I'm a reasonably competent researcher, but I found nothing tabulating suicide rates in nursing homes. There was a case of a man who killed his wife who had Alzheimer's and then turned the gun on himself, but that was in an assisted-living facility—where you have the ability to pack heat without the prying eyes of staff continually parading into the open door of your room. It's hard to kill yourself when you are under the close scrutiny—no matter how short-staffed—of the typical nursing home.

"How are you doing, Mr. Podolsky?"

"If I had a gun, I'd shoot myself."

Whatever I might think of Mr. Podolsky's right to shoot himself, I have an obligation to snitch on him. All therapists have a legal duty to warn (and violate confidences) if we determine a person is a danger to himself or others. If Mr. Podolsky had merely said, "If I woke up dead, I'd be happy," he would still be in the realm of passive suicidal ideation, and I would not have the duty to warn. When Mr. Podolsky formulates a plan—no matter how far-fetched—I walk back to the nursing station and have to report it.

"I hate to do this, but Mr. Podolsky says he wants to kill himself."

I hate to do it, because even though the nurses and I know a Podolsky suicide is highly unlikely, it means they have to put him on fifteen-minute checks—an aide peeks in, checks to see he's still alive, and makes a note of it in the chart. And the checks won't be discontinued until I or one of my colleagues certifies that Mr. Podolsky is no longer a potential danger to himself.

One of the few articles I found about suicidal behavior in nursing homes says it all in its title and brief abstract, "Suicide risk in frail elderly people relocated to nursing homes: In general, elders who consider suicide are over 85 years old, want to retain control of their lives, and have a high degree of self-esteem."

If I were to develop a theory of self-esteem, I'd put control or mastery at the top of the list. When my kids fib about having practiced the violin or refuse to do their homework, they are exerting control. When a prisoner in solitary confinement destroys everything in his cell—control. And when a nursing home resident expresses a desire to kill himself, it is an attempt to retain mastery of his immensely shrunken world. Today, I saw a resident, ninety-one, who is refusing his meds. They marked him down as noncompliant and demented. Rosofsky to the rescue, I found him certifiably noncompliant and certifiably nondemented.

Sometimes, I do a little good—retrieving someone from the scrap heap of dementia—that is, if anyone notices my evaluation.

"I don't need to take those pills to go to sleep, and if I don't want to, that's my business, none of theirs. If I want to lie awake all night tossing and turning, make them stop me." e. e. cummings understood this in his poem of a conscientious objector, "i sing of Olaf glad and big," when he has Olaf exclaim, "there is some shit I will not eat."

Although our lives are at least partly in thrall to our parents, our peers, and our genes, human contentment rests on at least the illusion of control and mastery. Perhaps that is what is encapsulated in Dutch euthanasia. It maintains the illusion of control. Don't have a gun? We'll hand you the drugs. Too disabled to pop the pills? Open your mouth and we'll pop them in for you.

In the United States, there is Oregon and its Death with Dignity

Act. This law does not go as far as the Dutch law, because it is limited to terminally ill patients. Intractable physical or psychic pain sufferers need not apply to die, as they can in the Netherlands. Oregon also doesn't allow your physician to assist you directly to die. The law simply allows your physician to prescribe lethal meds for you to take in the privacy of your own home—Socrates style, downing your hemlock with your disciples gathered around while you expound on the meaning of life as you descend into oblivion. You can go to the Oregon state government website and download the form—"Request for Medication to End My Life in a Humane and Dignified Manner"—to apply for the lethal dose. It's kind of a penultimate testament in which you certify that you are of sound mind—if not of body. The law is silent about people who cannot administer the dose to themselves, although no doctor need be present: "Open up, Mom. Here are your last meds." Something about me loves the fact that the website asks you to check with your health insurer to see whether this is a covered procedure. Covered procedure? You bet. Suicide is the ultimate cost saver for managed care.

For all the political fuss about this law, terminally ill people are not exactly beating down death's door to get their lethal meds. Since the law was enacted in 1997, a total of 292 patients have kicked the legal suicide bucket. In 2006, for example, under the provisions of the law, there were 46 deaths per 10,000—0.0046 percent. In contrast, 2 percent of deaths in the Netherlands fall under the provisions of its euthanasia law.

This does not mean the law is unpopular in Oregon. A state referendum to repeal it failed when 60 percent of the electorate voted to keep it on the books. Perhaps this means that people like the idea that they can end it if they really want to. Perhaps it means that it's harder to get something off the books than to get it on the books in the first place. Several other states have failed to pass physician-assisted suicide voter referendums. Others have failed to enact legislation, and a few State Supreme Courts have decided that physician-assisted suicide is unconstitutional—but not the United States Supreme Court. In 2006, by a 6–3 margin, it held that it was none of Attorney General John Ashcroft's legal business to interfere in a medical procedure. The Supremes ruled that it was up to the states, on an individual basis, to decide if you can get the hemlock prescription.

So if you are terminally ill in Oregon, and want to die, lucky you. But if you are not in Oregon, are you out of luck? Not necessarily. It's not as easy as buying crack on your local street corner, but it's not impossible to get the benefits of Oregon's law without being an Oregonian.

First, if you are capable, you can easily find ways to do yourself in. Suicide research is all over the map, but there is evidence that people with cancer or AIDS, for example, have a significantly higher suicide rate than those who don't. A study in Finland found that women and men with cancer were respectively 1.3 and 1.9 times more likely to kill themselves than the general population. In my own state of Connecticut, a survey found that although men with cancer were 2.3 times more likely to kill themselves than the general population, there was no increase in likelihood of suicide in women. These are not unremarkable numbers. People like the reassurance of knowing they can do it, even if they never pull the trigger.

If you are too cowardly or do not have the means or capability of killing yourself, there is a fair amount of bootleg physician-assisted suicide outside Oregon. In the neighboring state of Washington, a survey found that 26 percent of physicians had received a request for assisted suicide, and that two-thirds of the physicians receiving a request had granted the wish. Among AIDS physicians, the requests are dramatically higher. A survey of San Francisco physicians treating AIDS revealed that 98 percent had been asked for suicide assistance. On average, about 4 percent of the surveyed had granted such requests, and some physicians had granted dozens of requests.

Should we try to dissuade medically or psychically distressed people from killing themselves? There is the argument, against Szasz, that people who are depressed and receive treatment are likely to decide against suicide. This argument is worthy of consideration as long as we don't fall into the circular reasoning trap that anyone who wants to commit suicide is depressed.

In "Physician-Assisted Suicide: The Influence of Psychosocial Issues," published in the journal *Cancer Control* in 1999, an oncologist and a psychologist, William Breitbart, M.D., and Barry D. Rosenfeld, Ph.D., wrote that "many terminally ill patients are likely to be experiencing a depression that may be both treatable as well as temporary." "Temporary," of course, is a relative term when you are terminally ill, but Breitbart and Rosenfeld accept the idea that not all terminally ill people are depressed and that depression alone does not mean you are incapable of making a competent decision about your own death. They recommend the aggressive treatment of pain and depression, and then a reevaluation of whether the patient still wants to cash in his chips.

The recommendation for the aggressive treatment of depression, with the use of either meds or psychotherapy, does raise the questions of whether antidepressant medications could cloud your competent suicidal judgment and whether psychotherapy is merely a sophisticated way to talk you out of it. Because the diagnostic criteria for depression include a desire to end life, we have to be careful to exclude that as a criterion when an otherwise competent but suffering person requests assistance. And this reasoning leaves aside the deeper question of whether depression—even if we can validly think of it as an illness—can be an intractable illness, as intractable as severe physical pain, and be in itself the source of a reasonable desire to die. I've met some people for whom depression is a deeply embedded part of their being. People who have had every treatment imaginable—pills, psychotherapy, electric shock therapy—and want to end their suffering. Who am I to say no to them? To request them to spend some weeks, months, years talking to me instead?

"I'm depressed. I just want to end it," said Mr. Dolorean to me.

"Are you unhappy because you're sick and in this nursing home?"

"No. I've felt that way most of my life, but my obligations to my family kept me alive. Now they're all set, and I see no reason to go on here or anywhere else."

George Costanza said: "I love a good nap. Sometimes it's the only thing getting me out of bed in the mornings." Some people feel that way about life and the dirt nap.

After my father's phone call of death, I arrive at the nursing home, and he's lying in his bed, hooked up to an IV, all peaceful and quiet. No "Get the hell out of here!" I say, "Dad," and there's no response. I didn't expect one. I lay my hand on his arm, still warm and alive, his thin chest going up and down. They tell me the physician assistant has left the building, but the doctor is around, and he'll come and see my dad.

I sit in the uncomfortable plastic chair, flipping through the large-print *Reader's Digest*, glancing at my father, walking over to check he's still breathing. He doesn't have his dentures in, his mouth the pinched-hollow of the toothless. Little animation but the breathing.

After maybe a half-hour, the doc comes sauntering in. We know each other. He's the medical director. He does his doctor thing. Pokes and palpates. Listens through the stethoscope. Pulls up the eyelids.

"Is he going to die like your assistant said?"—me knowing that he will die but maybe not today.

"Hard to say. I've seen these old guys hang on for a while."

"What should we do?"

"Well, if you leave him here, he will die."

"So the hospital, then?"

"He'll live longer there, but recovery? I don't know," meaning: I doubt it.

I call Robert, and we opt for the hospital.

In addition to all the papers inside, the charts have stickers on the outside whose purpose is to say, Look here first before you do anything stupid.

For some residents these stickers warn of drug allergies—"No Penicillin!"—but more ubiquitous are "Full Code" or "DNR."

Full Code or Do Not Resuscitate—the lady or the tiger—expressing your or your legal guardian's wishes about your life and death.

Full Code means that if your heart or breathing stops, the medical staff will do everything they can to start your heart or your breathing—CPR, defibrillators, ventilators, IVs, feeding tubes. This is very expensive, and the chances of success when you're frail and old are slim. Even if they resuscitate successfully, you will likely wake up to a further diminished quality of life.

Robert and I had to make decisions.

Well before my father became certifiably incompetent, we had the prescience to obtain POA—power of attorney. Robert, on a trip to Florida, took Dad over to a local lawyer and in less than an hour we had the right to make medical and financial decisions. When he started spending his Social Security checks on get-rich-quick schemes, we had the legal power to work with his bank to put an end to it. Technically, Dad had the right to veto our moves, but he didn't make a fuss, because he had enough remaining sense to realize he needed to eat. Once Dad became incompetent, we were the automatic go-to guys for all medical decisions. If we weren't already POAs, given my father's incompetence, it would have been easy to be appointed by a court as conservators. But practically speaking, if you're the next of kin, even if you're not a conservator or POA, the doctors will defer to your wishes. It's only when family members with equal legal footing disagree among themselves that a mess could wind up in court. The courts have to break the tie.

So as a logician or lawyer would say, Robert and I or Robert or I decided not to let my father play out the string in his bare room at the nursing home but to resort to whatever remedies a hospital could provide.

We wondered whether we were going back on our directive not to resuscitate. Who knows where to draw the line? It wasn't like he had a heart attack. We weren't calling in the defibrillator infantry with the EMT cavalry close behind. Dad was just very, very—acutely as opposed to chronically—sick, and we were giving him a chance to get well—or as well as he could get.

Most of the charts I see have the DNR tags. Most people conclude there's no point in Full Code. Many, like my mother, plan ahead and have a living will that can be placed in the legal section of their charts. A living will has the ironic purpose of letting the testator die unmolested by medicine when the time comes.

The medical profession pushes DNR, not Full Code, for the nursing home set, although most of us youngsters walk through life with a presumption of Full Code. The average eighty-year-old male has a life expectancy of eight years; for females, it's ten. But for the frail and ill in the nursing home, longevity averages only two years. If you go into cardiac or pulmonary arrest, resuscitation adds only a few months to your life. If managed-care companies had complete control, they would probably make everyone DNR. It's more expensive to keep an old person alive than to let death take its natural course.

A paper by the Cornell University physician Haoming Qiu, "End of Life Care: The Cost of Living an Extra Year," published in the journal *The Triple Helix*, observes that "around 27 to 30 percent of Medicare payments go towards the 5 to 6 percent of Medicare beneficiaries who die in that year. Costs accelerate as the time of death approaches with costs in the final month of life accounting for 40 percent of the last year of life." Given these numbers, the cheapest way to die is to stay out of the hospital, or to leave it as soon as possible. Decision makers for countries with national health plans tend to think like decision makers for managed care companies, and they are making the hard decision to cut down on end-of-life costs. Qiu reasons, "Although each life is priceless, if the costs of keeping a dying person alive for one month can keep five young uninsured people healthy for ten years, then practicality dictates that we must utilize our resources where they will do the most good."

There are nonmonetary issues too—death with dignity, for one.

Do you want to peacefully take your leave? Or do you want your end to be a violent struggle—with fists pounding your chest, bolts of electricity through your body, tubes entering a hole cut through your throat? And if you survive that, do you want to be caught in a web of technology in an environment that defines sterile?

With a version of these thoughts in mind, I nevertheless wait for the ambulance to take my father to Saint Raphael's Hospital and then drive over to see him settled in. From his Army days, Dad knew about "Hurry up and wait," and it was hurry up and wait for death too. He was wheeled not directly up to a hospital room but into a cubicle in the emergency room. He lay there in his cubicle for hours, yet another curtain the sole means of privacy. The nurse told me they're waiting for a room, but I wonder if they're waiting to see if he'll live long enough to be worth a room. We were already running up the hospital expense meter, much more expensive than if we had left him in the nursing home, where he was hooked up to only one IV. Here there's the IV, plus various monitoring devices. The emergency room is high on tech and low on amenities. Behind his cot, I can watch a screen with real-time readouts of his heart rate, his breathing, his temperature—all up-and-down lines, no flat ones.

I walked over to the nursing station—banks of more monitors; somewhere there's one for Dad.

I ask the nurse, "How's he doing?"

"We're waiting for the attending to examine him."

I waited around for the attending—that is, the resident. As I was finishing off *The New York Times* crossword puzzle, he showed up, read the chart, looked at the monitor, did some laying of hands, and said there would be a room soon. He also called in the army—the kidney guy, the pulmonary guy, the cardiac guy. As yet, he doesn't have much to tell me except that Dad's not dead. I've noticed that too. It's okay to go home. They have my cell number, and I'm only ten minutes away.

At home there is something else waiting. Our thirteen-year-old dog, Aurora, can't stand up and get out of her doghouse. (I named her Aurora, because if you say it the right way it's a name a dog herself could say.) Aurora had been acting funny the past week—her head in a definite tilt following a fall on the stairs a few days before although, as with humans, we can't be sure whether the fall caused the head tilt or whether something underlying the head tilt caused the fall. But now she can't move, stares helplessly at nothing. Linda and I carry her to the car and drive her to the twenty-four-hour veterinary hospital. Aurora survives the night but the vet says long-term survival is unlikely. We could spend thousands to explore and operate, but Aurora is an old dog. Would she even survive the invasive diagnosis—let alone any possible cures? Linda gives me this grim update while I'm sitting next to Dad in his hospital room. With him, it's almost a miracle. He is sitting up and taking a bit of nourishment.

On the canine front, we euthanize Aurora. My wife gets that pleasure. I'm concentrating on the human, for now the easier task, sitting by my father watching TV, reading the paper, allowing solicitous nurses to bring me cups of coffee. It's Linda who gets to sit at the vet hospital when they give our poor, frail puppy—once a fierce beast—the needle, the executioner vet looking Linda in the eye and telling her, "You're doing the right thing," as she's bawling her eyes out, with my older son, eleven years old, alone just outside the room doing the same.

The calculus of euthanasia appears simpler for animals. Putting them out of their misery is as right for them as it is wrong for a human. We decline an individual burial for Aurora or even receiving her ashes. Her dust-to-dust remains will go into the general ash pile. I'm unsentimental. Am I uncaring? I seldom visit the graves of my parents—rationalizing that we Jews believe immortality is in memory; a grave works against living memory. I joke to Linda that after I'm buried, she'll turn to the assembled and say, "Now, that was sad, but what's for lunch?"

Aurora was gone but there's more. The next day, my mother-in-law feels sick. She says it's the heat. It's the heat, but the heat's in her. She's running a fever of 103. She walks slowly and painfully to my car, and it's another trip to the emergency room. After several hours—I'm shuttling up and down the elevator between my dad and Linda and her mom—she's admitted with a bladder infection. With our parents in the same hospital, and poor Aurora already a memory, Linda and I can consolidate our trips. Very efficient.

In only a few days, Helen is doing better and will soon be discharged, while my father, who appeared to have rallied, is slipping away toward his ending.

I hate to jump ahead in this story and give you a spoiler, but if this were a country-and-western song written when this was happening in 2003, I might have named it "My Dog and Daddy Died, but My Mother-in-Law Survived." And to spoil it even more, three years later Helen was back in the hospital with pneumonia. She survived the pneumonia, but being in a hospital exposes you to a variety of infections, in her case *Clostridium difficile*—C. diff, *très difficile*.

One of her doctors, a surly fellow, who talked to you as if he were doing you a favor rather than providing a service, admitted in an unguarded moment that C. diff was "running rampant in the hospital." It's not a fun way to go, with GI unpleasantries like diarrhea and nausea. C. diff is taking its place alongside staph as one of the superbugs you will be reading about in tabloid headlines and medical thrillers. A CDC report indicated that C. diff infections grew fivefold from 1999 to 2004. No surprise, since it is resistant to antibiotics and finds a fertile playing field in hospitals.

During her later hospitalization, Helen agreed to move from her home of fifty years to a nearby assisted-living center with Long Island Sound views, but she didn't get to enjoy that much, spending most of her time sick and in a nursing home. We remained hopeful that she would make it out of the nursing home, but she continued to slowly but inexorably go downhill. One day, I'm on the interstate and my cell phone rings. It's the social worker at Helen's nursing home. She's apologetic for calling me.

"I couldn't reach Linda, but Helen just passed away."

Surprised but not shocked, I pull into a rest area so I can concentrate, undistracted by driving, on a call to Linda.

Unobserved by us, the men in dark suits and a somber expression come to take Helen away. When she reappears, Linda asks me to take photos of Helen lying in state at her wake—something of a family tradition. They reside not on the nineteenth-century mantel with all our other ancestors, but on the twenty-first-century family computer in the same folder with my kids frolicking at Christo's Gates in Central Park.

My father takes a further turn for the worse. He's delirious on top of his dementia. (As an aside, notice how many of the negative words begin with *d*—a theme for a philologist: delirious, dysphagic, depression, disease, dementia, death. What a downer.) Delirium is a kind of temporary dementia. It can be caused by drunkenness (another *d* word) or disease. Many elderly people with infections—such as pneumonia, bladder infections, urinary tract infections—develop symptoms similar to dementia. If a resident suddenly acts demented, checking for an infection is the first thing to do. This is the origin of the expression "delirious from the fever." At age eight, I had pneumonia. I was delirious for three days, and I remember the pervasive odor of coconuts. I retain to this day an aversion to anything coconut. A few years ago, my mother had pneumonia, delirious too, in the hospital for three days. Fully regaining her mind, she had no memory of it. Whenever my group sees a resident just out of the hospital, we caution the staff to wait a couple of weeks before consigning the person to the dementia diagnosis or, worse still, the dementia ward. But in my poor father's case, delirium is a clouding of consciousness on top of an already clouded consciousness.

Dysphagia, inability to swallow, is common in nursing homes and the geriatric population. It can be caused by damage to the various muscles involved in swallowing. It is also associated with Parkinson's disease, strokes, brain injuries, and cancer. All these are present in the nursing home, but many of the dysphagia cases are associated primarily with dementia—eventually reaching that point where food is not recognized as food and the idea of swallowing is not part of whatever consciousness remains.

The problem with dysphagia, whether physical or cognitive, is that the food, instead of going down to your tummy, could wind up in your lung—aspiration—and provide a breeding ground for pneumonia bacteria. A speech pathologist—yet another nursing home consultant—working in conjunction with a dietitian, evaluates your dysphagia. You might go to pureed food. You might be in the feeding program—staff nurturingly spooning pabulum into your mouth, and watching you swallow. It's back to high chair days, but you're in a wheelchair. I don't know if they say as they raise the spoon, "Open up, Mr. Jones. Here's comes the train into the tunnel."

In my father's comatose case, the options were slim and none.

Slim meant a feeding tube. Before World War I, prison authorities inserted tubes through the nostrils or mouths of British suffragettes on hunger strikes, and worked them down into their stomachs before pouring food into them. Quite painful, but it didn't hurt fostering sympathy for the right to vote. Almost a century later, the United States has been doing the same to hunger strikers at Guantánamo Bay—their hands and legs tied for hours, food tubes fully inserted.

The venerably designed nasogastric feeding tube, whether for forced or therapeutic feeding, is a temporary solution. It would be a logistical nightmare to have to insert them every day. For my father, there would have been a tube permanently emplaced through his stomach wall—variously called the G-tube or PEG tube. First, they would sedate him. Then they would snake an endoscope with a powerful light on its end down his esophagus to the stomach. The light is powerful enough so that it can be seen through the stomach wall as if X—the light—marks the spot where you cut a hole in the abdomen and insert the feeding tube into the stomach. Once the tube is in place, you insert gruel at the outside end and it slides right into the stomach—no tasting, no swallowing, no mastication, no savoring. This can be a lifesaver for alert and oriented cancer patients or for people with damaged or missing jaws or esophagi. In my father's case—compromised more in mind than in body—he would likely try to pull out the tube if he were awake. Very bloody, so he would be sedated and physically restrained. Sedated, restrained, with food inserted directly into the stomach. Nice life, eh?

And there's this catch. Had Robert and I agreed to insert the tube, it would have been hell to take it out. The medical-ethical logic is that it's okay not to initiate a life-sustaining procedure, but once you proactively sustain a life, to unsustain it—to remove a feeding tube—would be illegal physician-assisted suicide. Faced with this dilemma it's no wonder there is the occasional case of a husband literally pulling the plug on a lingering wife, or the more grisly murder-suicide. So in the end we opted for no chance, no feeding, over slim chance, feeding tube, with the doctors assuring us that starving to death is painless, as they say it is for lobsters in boiling water.

With the decision not to feed Dad, we revisit the Alaskan nomads moving on, leaving Old Koskoosh alone as the wolves draw nearer.

And with that, the hospital has nothing more to do.

As I walk through many a nursing home, I pass people who are hanging on by a thread, IVs, breathing tubes, PEG tubes, tanks of oxygen. Some will be that way for months or years, and some are close to the ritualistic pronouncement of death, followed by the call to the funeral, and finalized with the last mandated documentation for the chart.

No doctor is necessary; another sticker usually reads "RN May Pronounce."

There is undeniable relief when you accept the end. But life clings. Lichenous life clings to rocks in the Antarctic. Complex systems of life sport around deep-sea thermal vents that spew out water heated to 600 degrees. Human life is everywhere and overcomes obstacles I can only imagine—from abused youth who grow to love and nurture their own children to old residents in nursing homes missing body parts, tethered to technology, greeting me with a smile.

And there's Dad's continuing weeks after the announcement of his imminent demise—life's last gasp—going out with neither a bang nor a whimper, his fingers hanging on to a cliff's edge as death stomps on his hands. As Jimmy Durante—I watched him regularly with my mother—sang, "Did you ever have the feeling you wanted to go, and still have the feeling you wanted to stay?"

Dad's systems were shutting down one by one, lights in a candelabrum winking out, the room growing darker. I did not want Dad's final days to be in a nursing home of which I already had a low opinion. But there was an option: the hospice. The first U.S. hospice, in fact.

Places called hospices appeared on the pilgrim trails early in the middle ages. On the road to the remains of Saint James, disciple of Jesus, in Spain—El Camino de Santiago—institutions sprang up devoted to hospitality for pilgrims, many of whom were seeking a miracle cure for incurable illnesses. Later, hospices, precursors of hospitals, were founded specifically to provide care for the sick and the dying. The modern hospice movement was founded in England by a nurse, Cicely Saunders. While caring for David Tasma in 1944—a Jewish Warsaw Ghetto escapee who was dying of cancer, cut off from family, friends, and home—the two discussed the idea of an institution, a hospice, for the dying. Tasma left Saunders five hundred pounds for the purpose, "I'll be a window in your home." Nineteen years later, after study, caring for the dying, and becoming a physician, Saunders established St. Christopher's Hospice in London. She wrote: "The name hospice, 'a resting place for travelers or pilgrims', was chosen because this will be something between a hospital and a home, with the skills of one and the hospitality, warmth, and the time of the other." In 1965, around the time Elisabeth Kübler-Ross was writing *On Death and Dying,* Saunders came to Yale as a visiting professor and spread the word to us colonials.

One outcome of her visit was the Connecticut Hospice, founded in 1974—where Dad would go. In the beginning, the hospice focused on visits by nurses and volunteers to patients dying at home. It is probably more than a coincidence that the hospice movement took root about the same time some expectant mothers elected to have their deliveries at home attended by midwives—another throwback. People were getting tired of doing everything in an institution. This was the time when labor and delivery while remaining conscious became the norm in hospitals. Fathers were in the room, not smoking and pacing somewhere else. Not dying in the hospital was in the zeitgeist. The stark, sterile environment infused with technology was losing its charm. People wanted to be like my grandmother—be born and die in a bed at home.

Eventually the Connecticut Hospice, recognizing that not everyone had the desire or the means to die at home, established an in-patient facility in Branford, Connecticut.

Hospice care, whether in-house or at home is palliative care. It provides comfort for the patient, "easing symptoms without providing a cure," when there is irreversible illness. It's a mixture of pain management, counseling, and plain old handholding. It even comes into the nursing home. Next to stickers for Full Code or DNR, I sometimes see Hospice Care. This means that the care of a dying resident is now directed by the hospice team that comes into the nursing home—another set of outside consultants.

Now I don't mean to be cynical about this—although if you have read this far you know it's hard for me to help myself—but this is a big moneymaker, fully reimbursable by Medicare. This is not new. The original hospices on El Camino de Santiago were about Mammon as well as God. The hospitality was free, but gratuities were freely accepted. The notables who established the hospices were possibly more interested in earthly than heavenly reward—although with paid indulgences, heavenly reward in those days had a much more tangible feel to it than today. The hospices were an economic stimulus. Around them sprouted inns, shops, and brothels. They were the seed of more than one town. Beyond the immediate environs, an infrastructure of roads and bridges developed to serve this incipient tourist industry.

The Connecticut Hospice loves its volunteers—"nobility of character and gentleness of soul"—but takes the shape of a medical institution easily recognizable to me. It is a nonprofit, a slippery concept. Yale–New Haven Hospital is a nonprofit, but I see its advertising billboards lining the highway alongside ads for motels, McDonald's, and adult lingerie.

At the hospice, there is the usual cast of medical characters. In an elocution that could serve as advertising copy for my own geriatric-services company, I see on their website: "Like a tapestry woven with many different threads, care by The Connecticut Hospice, Inc. is an interplay of the skills of so many different professions. Within hospice home and inpatient care, physicians, nurses, pharmacists, social workers, clergy, artists, volunteers, and consultants actively assist each patient and family in resolving the myriad of difficulties surrounding irreversible illness. It is the 'team' approach—comprehensive, coordinated palliative care without gaps or overlaps—that truly distinguishes hospice within the health care system."

Team approach means that we have a job for every possible professional who can bill Medicare. Nobility of character is reserved for the nonreimbursable volunteers. There are doctors, nurses, social workers, dieticians, and recreational therapists, and on the outpatient side, the home-care that visits nursing homes—just like me.

I ask the same question about this place as I do about the nursing home: Why does it have to look and act like a hospital to do what it has to do?

It's a Thursday, the day before Dad would be transferred, and I pay a visit. I know the road, a few miles up the shoreline from where Linda grew up. For years, driving down this road—which winds its way eventually to the Post Road with its strip malls, fast-food restaurants, and gas stations—a mile or so after the beach with the view of the Thimble Islands, I'd pass the sign pointing to the hospice and not give much thought to it aside from a vague awareness of its being some kind of well-known historical institution. This time, I turn right at the hospice sign and wind up on a parcel of valuable waterfront property—looking out to the same Thimble Islands—a Hamptons for the rich and famous and reclusive.

Unbeknownst to Dad, he's approaching his ninetieth birthday, which would be July 19, 2003. When he turned eighty, still in reasonable control of his faculties, he told me, "Eighty is nothing. Ninety is something." It's July, typically warm and humid. Here, in contrast to other nursing home–type places, I see a couple of beds with patients in them rolled right down to the water's edge for the view. But when I walk inside it's all familiar. The nursing station, the two to a room with a curtain for privacy. I'll try not to judge this book by its cover.

I go back to a place I've already passed judgment on to pick up a couple of things, and Dad's room is empty. It's as if he never lived there. I walk over to the nursing station.

"What happened in my father's room? There's nothing there!"

"We moved his stuff out when we heard he was going to hospice."

"But there's nobody in his room. You couldn't wait?"

I'm raising my voice.

"You're disturbing the other residents."

I could say something lamely clever like, "You're disturbing me," but rage does not mix with cleverness.

"I care no less for the other residents than you do. His body is still warm and you're kicking him out. You could have called me! You had my number."

"We're going to have to ask you to leave."

This is their answer to my question about not calling me to pick up my father's stuff. In their minds, they're following the regulations, and customer service isn't one of them.

I get a grip, and I wait downstairs in the lobby. They're going to bring me his stuff.

Down the hall, I hear someone pushing a flat-bed cart. There are four cardboard boxes. My father's earthly remains. All eighty-nine years distilled into something that fits easily into the back of my minivan. There are his clothes, most of which we bought for him from the Small Man's Shop, the *Reader's Digest*s, his CDs minus the stolen CD player, a toothbrush—his legacy.

And that's it for Dad's nursing home. I've never set foot into it again, never driven by it, but I find it hard—as you have seen—to tweak it every chance I get. This is the toned-down version. Having a book to write gives you a place to store your enemies for eternity. Dante had the best writing gig—never off-topic for him to put whomever he wanted in the Inferno. I have to make do with Dad's nameless nursing home.

The next morning, Friday, July 11, 2003—a little more than a week before his ninetieth birthday—they move Dad to the hospice. Will he make it there? I drive over. Dad's still as quiet as a mouse. The room is quiet too. Unlike the nursing homes the hospice resembles, it's all very hushed. There's a roommate, if that's the right word. They're not side by side as in the typical nursing home, but facing each other. Everybody is asleep or possibly comatose. Everyone on the edge of the same cliff as Dad, all lined up, hanging on now by their fingertips alone.

I walk over to the window. I can hardly see the water through all the summer foliage. Outside it's lush and alive.

A cute young thing (something I never fail to notice), a nice Jewish girl I see by her name tag, comes in.

"Hi, I'm Naomi, the social worker. Let me know if you need anything or just want to talk."

"Thank you. I'm fine."

The tables are turned. I'm the client—even if she has read the chart and knows what I do for a living—I wonder if she's relieved I won't present much work for her. One less burden for the caseload. I wonder about her job, when you know that everyone is going to die—not in some indeterminate future, but quite soon. Freud said the only possible advantage physicians have in becoming analysts is they are used to death, and, thereby, failure. No problem for Naomi. I've joked that the way this book ends is that everybody dies. It's not a surprise ending for Naomi. She aces the analyst entrance exam.

I go home and take a nap. It could be a long night. Could be the deathwatch. It's all up to me. My kids need their mother. My brother is hours away, and he's made the trip more than once in the past few weeks. He'll come on the weekend.

I bring a book. I always have something to read. As a child, I would pick up wrappers on the street and read them. At one time I could recite verbatim every word of the Rice Krispies box, circa 1952. Now it's 2003; I doubt my father imagined he would meet his end in Branford, Connecticut, having lived most of his life in Brooklyn, with a detour to Europe to slog through the mud and blood of World War II, before joining his brethren in West Palm Beach, Florida—less of a journey than his parents made from Pinsk, Belarus.

The book I bring to the bedside is the recently published *Harry Potter and the Order of the Phoenix*. It's the fifth in the series, the one with longing for family, underscored by the death of Sirius Black, Harry's godfather. Perhaps Naomi would disapprove of someone bringing a book to attend a parent's death, but that's modern life, and like me, she has probably seen everything. When I woke up after eight hours of surgery, two things let me know I was possibly okay. In the recovery room, I could move my left arm, the one on the side of the tumor. Later, they wheeled me into a regular hospital room and my favorite show, *Jeopardy!*, was on the TV. (I've qualified three times to be a contestant, but maybe they don't like the looks of me, never having called me to be on the show.) I don't remember the question, but I nailed Final Jeopardy. I imagine myself at my own dying, the TV on, wondering if I'll make it to the end of the show. Now I'm facing Dad's final jeopardy by his side.

Across the room, there are a few visitors with Dad's roommate. It's still light as they leave the patient and one man—a bit younger than me—behind. The two of us step in the hall and have a companionable chat. Some years ago, we would have been lighting each other's cigarettes to go with the cups of coffee we're holding. Strangers when we meet, we have dying fathers in common.

"It's amazing how these old guys hold on," he tells me.

I concur with my tale of Dad's sentence to imminent death weeks ago. The man tells me of his three brothers, all married with children. He's the never married one who has lived with his father all his life, including the past two years and the battle with cancer. Something in me envies their comfortable relationship. But I also feel sad for him. His whole life, his father, soon to be gone. What will he go home to? I get to go home to the *Sturm und Drang* of domestic tranquillity.

He bids me a good evening and goes home to his already empty rooms. The nurse comes by and, after checking Dad's vital signs, looks me in the eye and says, "I don't think you should go home. There's probably not much time left."

And I thought there could be the weekend for Robert to join me, but it's all me—me and my dad.

I sit by the bed, while the nurse draws the curtain—the final curtain—around us, open my book, unable to concentrate, listen to Dad's breathing, not much of anything on my mind. He's already in oblivion, has been in oblivion, and now he's going to die.

It's around nine p.m.—getting dark at the end of a long summer's day—and Dad's breathing sounds different, like gravel shaking in a paper bag. Is this the death rattle? I call for the nurse, who arrives armed with a stethoscope. She listens to his heart.

"He's gone," and she leaves us behind again. Dry-eyed, heartless me, I cry mostly for dead animals. I kiss dead Dad on his still warm forehead, as if it's expected of me, as if someone is looking, although nobody, unless you count God, is watching. But I'm in part a good Jew. Whatever I may or may not feel, I've done my duty. Kant and the Torah would approve. It's a mitzvah. I abandoned no one. But after sitting there for a while, wondering about what thoughts should be in my mind, I drive home to my family.

My mother—dead already at the time for five years—would likely resent my father's getting to rest near me in New Haven, while she is somewhat far off in Montefiore Cemetery in Queens, New York. But she's with her family—along with Rabbi Menachem Schneerson, the Messiah of the Lubavitcher Hasidim, and the artist Barnett Newman, whose gravestone replicates in granite the blank slate of his paintings. Dad will rest alone among strangers. I'll likely not join him. His small Jewish cemetery is close to full, and my temple will be sending my body to its new suburban location.

There's little time for maudlin reflection. We Jews bury the next day, except in my father's case we skip Saturday, the Sabbath, for a Sunday burial. No one will have to miss work. I'd already made the preparations in advance with the funeral director—even to the point of arranging a military guard of honor, to which Dad is entitled as a veteran.

Sunday morning, our little band of mourners heads for the cemetery. Dad's blood relatives in attendance number seven—his two sons, and his five grandchildren. Along with our wives, there are some in-laws. There are two soldiers. They drove down from Fort Drum in New York, 319 miles to New Haven, truly a kindness of strangers. Later they will decline to come over to the house for a bite, anticipating their five-hour drive back to base. We walk the short distance in this postage-stamp-size cemetery to the graveside, where the rabbi gives his well-conceived but secondhand memorial, nothing to blame him for, his notes are based on the hearsay of my brother and me. It's about my dad's service to his country and his love of family. The grave is near a fence separating the cemetery from an apartment complex. I hear a dog barking, and a woman yelling at the dog to shut up. All falls quiet, though, as my older son picks up his trumpet and "Taps" cuts through the heavy morning air.

A nice touch. I couldn't be prouder. Maybe I cry not only for animals but for children too.

During my brief professorial career, I likened the student body to a river running through it. The river always young, always the same age while I would grow older. Working with the elderly, I'm well downstream now, yet the river of life still flows past. They're all the same age again as they flow past me again, but they're older, and I'm catching up to them too. As Swinburne, another aficionado of death and decay, wrote in "The Garden of Proserpine," "even the weariest river winds somewhere safe to sea."

Death used to be the great equalizer, but today we get a jump on Mr. D. The nursing home, death's antechamber, imposes a kind of predeceased uniformity on us with its standard-issue rooms, and its standard-issue routines. All this while we're quite alive.

It's easy to think that having children is your ticket to immortality. Your genes in the gene pool. But my children remind me of my mortality too, that the arc of their narrative will extend far beyond my more limited future, even farther than if I had had them younger in my own life. I had my children late, not Tony Randall late, but late enough so that they're only in their adolescence as I approach Social Security. As these things go, my health is excellent, but when I stumble, I'm old enough to wonder if this is the start of some deficit and decline. I feel bad not about my neck but about my shoulder. It hurts, and there's an inoperable tumor dormant but alive.

Thinking of my not totally horrible but less than idyllic childhood, I can joke that having children later in life means you won't be a burden on them when they're middle-aged. But I can regret knowing I'll likely not see my grandchildren wed, and possibly won't even meet any grandchildren at all.

My youngest child will be my age in the 2060s. If he lives long and the world still exists, he could survive to the twenty-second century and live in three different centuries—surely, his own children could be alive then. I like to point out that Bertrand Russell, who was alive and well in his nineties when I was an adult, had John Stuart Mill, born 1806, as his godfather. Mill's godfather was another philosopher, Jeremy Bentham, born 1748. Viewing time and history this way, only a few degrees of separation can bridge centuries looking both backward and forward.

Yet it's all finite. Everyone who was my age when I was born is now dead. The population has completely turned over. We can luck out with genes and take good care of ourselves and survive perhaps a decade or two beyond average life expectancy, but when you're dead, you're dead forever (afterlife, resurrection, and reincarnation aside). I know I can be flippant about these things, but the thought of my death stands my hair on end and sends a chill feeling down my spine—my prefrontal lobes communicating with my reptilian brain. I look down at my typing hands and know that the gold ring around my finger will someday circle my bony skeletal remains. Humans have the gift of consciousness—protoplasm having become aware of itself. Along with the gift of the awareness of being is the curse of the knowledge of our end. Oblivion is the destination of the stoic's cart, on which we choose to ride or be dragged behind. If I had intractable pain, I could imagine wishing for death; otherwise, I hope to be dragged over the edge.

Writing this book is my Hail Mary pass at an obituary in *The New York Times* or even just the local paper. It's daunting to see how meager the manuscript is. The computer file for the whole book is no bigger than a workaday snapshot from my digital camera. It alone probably won't get me the obit, and I can lament not focusing sooner on being a writer, grabbing fame with a long output of books. But even with Shakespeare, no one more famous, I can hold everything he wrote in the palm of one hand. I know that's the wrong way to look at it, that Shakespeare lives throughout the space of our infinite minds—and I will occupy only a minuscule portion of that. If you are reading this, I have reached out to you from my comfortable obscurity. That is an achievement. But living on in memory—no matter how soaring that sounds—is only another way of saying you're dead.

Everyone understands this, and there is a kind of comfort in knowing we all die. This is the comfort of Buddhism, all merging with the Great Soul, or of Hasidism, all of us a spark from the Great Light. We can get solace from such thinking even if it's not true.

And I can still take comfort from my children, as alike and different from each other as they are alike and different from me.

Before my daughter became the "world is too much with her late and soon" jaded adolescent self, the subject of mortality came up, and she said, "Can't we talk about puppies and ponies instead?" before realizing with a shudder that puppies and ponies die too. The shock of mortality is the first end of innocence.

My older son, a wisecracker like me, tells me I have to be nice to him. "I'm going to pick out your nursing home."

I hope not.

After a forgettably minor offense, I joked to my younger son—who understands time and numbers—that I'd be grounding him for the rest of his life.

"No, Dad. You'll be grounding me for the rest of your life."

I hope so.

AFTERWORD

Richard Nixon supposedly said, "Honesty is not always the best policy, but sometimes it's worth a try." In recent years, the honesty of personal histories has come under increasing scrutiny. Several memoir writers have exaggerated or fabricated details of their lives and have suffered scorn—if not poverty—for their efforts. For the layperson, there is no law mandating truth, but the reader of memoirs expects at least a try at honesty. The medical professional who writes about patients has the paradoxically opposite obligation—fiction. We have to protect the confidentiality of our patients. HIPAA mandates that dishonesty is the best policy. There is a range of opinion about how to achieve this. At one extreme, some advocate written consent from any patient who is the object of a writing exercise. Even if consent is granted, there still is the obligation to disguise patients so they cannot be identified by either the casual or the meticulous reader. In the case of writing about elderly residents of nursing homes, obtaining consent was not a practical possibility. I met many of the people I write about years ago, often for only a brief encounter. Many are deceased. To meet my ethical obligations to them, I relied on a variety of strategies to protect their identities and privacy. The patients in this book do not represent real people. Any resemblance to a particular person is accidental, inadvertent, and unintended. I have no doubt that some might read this book and say, "This is me," even if it isn't. I would count such recognition as artistic success, and evidence that I have provided an accurate representation of the life and times of our elders. As the psychologists Clyde Kluckhorn and Henry Murray wrote more than sixty years ago, "Every man is in certain respects like all other men, like some other men, and like no other men."

Professional responsibilities aside, when writing about my personal life, the only impediment to exactness is the frailty of my memory.

ACKNOWLEDGMENTS

There are many to thank for this book, but I want to pay particular note to the following:

From idea to book it has been a long journey, and, my wife, Linda, never wavered in her support. In fact, she calmly—no matter my pessimism—assumed it would happen.

My agent, John F. Thornton, picked my proposal off the so-called slush pile. Without his expertise and counsel, this book would not have happened.

My editor, Jeff Galas, instantly saw the potential and patiently and insightfully shepherded the project into publication.

Megan Newman, Avery publisher, agreed with Jeff that this was a task worth doing.

Special gratitude to all the people living within and without the eldercare system who inspired this book, and to their caregivers—both family and professionals—who toil tirelessly, and often thanklessly.